For my father, Desmond Daniel MacMahon (1933-2006), who for some reason took me to that squishy green track at St. Joseph's High School in Metuchen, New Jersey, when I was eight years old to run one lap around the track with all the boys. My older sister was running a race that day, but for some reason I was thrown into the mix. When the starter pistol went off, I ran as fast as I could, which was all I knew to do. I was not a runner at the start of that race, but I have been a runner ever since.

And for my mother, Nancy MacMahon (1935-2022), who somehow made it to all of my meets in high school and who began exercising regularly during her late 40s and for the rest of her life. Talking to her after finishing my first 100-mile race in 2015, she said to me, "I didn't want to do my morning workout today, but I thought of you—out there all day and all night and into this morning—and thought, *If Caolan can do that, I can do my workout.*"

They did not always understand what I was doing, but they always supported me and at times showed a deep understanding of how much it means to me.

CONTENTS

Foreword   vii

Preface   ix

Acknowledgments   xiii

PART I   RUNNING

1 Run by Your Own Rules: Understanding Realities Are Not Restrictions   3

2 Find Your Drive: Determining Goals and Creating Habits   21

3 Adapt to Change: Addressing the Needs of Female Runners   35

PART II   TRAINING

4 Identifying the Building Blocks of Successful Training   49

5 Establishing and Maintaining an Aerobic Base   63

6 Maximizing Training While Minimizing Injury   73

7 Incorporating Rest and Recovery   97

RUNNING PAST 50

Your Guide to Running Longevity and Success

Caolan MacMahon

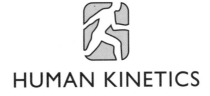

Library of Congress Cataloging-in-Publication Data

Names: MacMahon, Caolan, 1963- author.
Title: Running past 50 : your guide to running longevity and success / Caolan MacMahon.
Other titles: Running past fifty
Description: Champaign, IL : Human Kinetics, 2025. | Includes bibliographical references.
Identifiers: LCCN 2024022341 (print) | LCCN 2024022342 (ebook) | ISBN 9781718213944 (paperback) | ISBN 9781718213951 (epub) | ISBN 9781718213968 (pdf)
Subjects: LCSH: Running for older people. | Running--Training.
Classification: LCC GV1061.18.A35 M33 2025 (print) | LCC GV1061.18.A35 (ebook) | DDC 796.42071--dc23/eng/20240730
LC record available at https://lccn.loc.gov/2024022341
LC ebook record available at https://lccn.loc.gov/2024022342

ISBN: 978-1-7182-1394-4 (print)

Copyright © 2025 by Caolan MacMahon

Human Kinetics supports copyright. Copyright fuels scientific and artistic endeavor, encourages authors to create new works, and promotes free speech. Thank you for buying an authorized edition of this work and for complying with copyright laws by not reproducing, scanning, or distributing any part of it in any form without written permission from the publisher. You are supporting authors and allowing Human Kinetics to continue to publish works that increase the knowledge, enhance the performance, and improve the lives of people all over the world.

To report suspected copyright infringement of content published by Human Kinetics, contact us at **permissions@hkusa.com**. To request permission to legally reuse content published by Human Kinetics, please refer to the information at **https://US.HumanKinetics.com/pages/permissions-translations-faqs**.

This publication is written and published to provide accurate and authoritative information relevant to the subject matter presented. It is published and sold with the understanding that the author and publisher are not engaged in rendering legal, medical, or other professional services by reason of their authorship or publication of this work. If medical or other expert assistance is required, the services of a competent professional person should be sought.

Senior Acquisitions Editor: Michelle Earle; **Senior Developmental Editor:** Laura Pulliam; **Managing Editors:** Hannah Werner, Kim Kaufman; **Copyeditor:** Erica Warren; **Indexer:** Rebecca L. McCorkle; **Graphic Designer:** Denise Lowry; **Cover Designer:** Keri Evans; **Cover Design Specialist:** Susan Rothermel Allen; **Photograph (cover):** Kingfisher Productions/DigitalVision/Getty Images; **Photo Asset Manager:** Laura Fitch; **Photo Production Manager:** Jason Allen; **Senior Art Manager:** Kelly Hendren; **Illustrations:** © Human Kinetics; **Printer:** Versa Press

Human Kinetics books are available at special discounts for bulk purchase. Special editions or book excerpts can also be created to specification. For details, contact the Special Sales Manager at Human Kinetics.

Printed in the United States of America   10 9 8 7 6 5 4 3 2 1

The paper in this book is certified under a sustainable forestry program.

Human Kinetics
1607 N. Market Street
Champaign, IL 61820
USA

United States and International
Website: **US.HumanKinetics.com**
Email: info@hkusa.com
Phone: 1-800-747-4457

Canada
Website: **Canada.HumanKinetics.com**
Email: info@hkcanada.com

E8682

PART III PROGRAMMING

8 Creating Your Training Plan — 111

9 5K, 10K, and Half-Marathon Training Plans — 121

10 Marathon and Ultramarathon Training Plans — 139

11 Transitional Training Plans — 157

PART IV COMPETING

12 Preparing to Compete — 167

13 Designing Your Race-Day Strategy — 181

14 Staying Focused and Avoiding Setbacks — 193

Bibliography 201

Index 204

About the Author 210

FOREWORD

Caolan and I both love running races of all distances, but we're especially fond of marathons and ultramarathons. The only race experiences we seem to have in common, however, are a few Boston Marathons. If ever there were a race that made two runners feel like kindred spirits, the 2018 Boston Marathon was the one: 40-degree temperatures, headwinds of 30 miles per hour, and torrential rain pummeling the course throughout the race. We'll be forever bonded by surviving that experience.

When Caolan asked me to write a foreword to her book *Running Past 50*, our shared experiences made it feel like I was doing a favor for an old friend, even though we have never actually met. I definitely qualify as a member of the book's target audience! I didn't run my first race until I was 57, so my entire running career (18 years and counting) fits into that category. I was hoping that reading this book would teach an old dog new tricks. I did have a few tricks up my sleeve—having set 35 national and world records—but I was eager to discover what additional lessons Caolan had in store for me.

Right away, Caolan grabbed my attention by articulating many thoughts about running that I have never been able to put into words. And she kept pulling that same trick over and over as the first chapter unfolded. As I read further into the book, I was pleased to discover that not only was there much for me to learn, but there was also much for nearly anybody to learn—not just those over 50. I often found myself thinking that it should be titled *Running Without a Coach*, but even that is too limiting! I do have a coach, and when I'm asked about my training, I respond that I just do what my coach tells me to do. Yet that isn't really true. Having a coach is not a one-way street. A good coach relies on feedback from the client, and this book gives readers a much better grasp of how to communicate as you progress.

So, who is this book really for? It will be most useful to those interested in coaching themselves. Setting goals, structuring workouts, specific workouts—it's all in there. But even if you do have a coach, you will still learn much about how to train and run.

I now find myself at a tricky point in my running career. I still want to run a lot of races, I still hope to set national and world records, and I still want to have a lot of fun. But I'm starting to feel *old*, and I can no longer do it all. This book is helping me with this transition and especially in setting realistic goals and adjusting my training to accommodate new routines.

—Gene Dykes

PREFACE

Why do you run? Why do so many older folks come into the sport of running later in life? Why do so many older runners continue to pursue the sport into their 50s, 60s, 70s, and even beyond? Those in the grand-master and senior-grand-master age groups are a fairly new phenomenon, venturing into largely uncharted territories. As such, they are still the object of study and speculation as they push the frontiers of possibility.

> Running is a must if you want to live, not just exist.
>
> *Joe Vigil*

This book is for all you who wish to keep running, exploring, discovering, and achieving with no end in sight. It's for all who wish to continue living on your own terms, based not on preconceived notions of what it is to be older but rather on passionate desires that have yet to be quenched. This book is for you who are grateful for the endurance, power, and strength you possess. It's for you who still yearn for those 20-something personal bests and seek new, exciting challenges. This book is for all you who just enjoy running and want to keep doing it for the rest of your lives.

But let's be honest: A lot of people out there will tell you to stop being so silly. They'll say you can't do this forever, which is an obviously true statement—it just may not be true yet. I have had my share of friends, family, and even doctors tell me that I should stop all this running stuff. But I don't want to, and I don't have to.

I began running when I was eight years old. I ran throughout my childhood, adolescence, and young adulthood. Running has been a part of my identity for most of my life. When I was in my mid-20s, the road-racing scene drew me in and held me tight. But then, after several years of relentlessly pursuing ever more ambitious 10K times (that's what everyone raced in the '80s and early '90s), I quit, in an instant, right before my 27th birthday. I affectionately refer to this episode as my "first midlife crisis." I was so burned out due to perfectionistic tendencies and very lofty goals, both resulting in too much pressure. I grew to hate racing, but I still loved running.

I continued to run for hours upon hours every week, watchless and free. Running remained a necessary part of my daily life. I needed to run as much as I needed to breathe. In 1993, when I was 30, I ran one marathon, the Maine Marathon, just because I wanted to. I didn't do any extra training other than adding several long runs, but I found that those long runs got in the way of weekend camping and climbing trips, so I never ran another marathon. I always told myself I would run another one when I was old and done climbing seriously. Someday I would run in New York, but that would have to wait for later.

Then in 2008, I sustained my first running injury in years. Several months of physical therapy with no improvement led me to an MRI to rule out a meniscus tear. The results were grim beyond anything I could have imagined at that point in my life.

The nurse practitioner (NP) who examined me called with the results.

NP: "We have the MRI results. You have significant osteoarthritis. I know you don't want to hear this, but you won't be able to run anymore. I would encourage you to try biking."

Me: "Um. What are you saying? What can be done?"

NP: "Nothing can be done. You're too young for a knee replacement."

And in a matter of seconds, my life had changed. All those plans of "someday when I'm old" vanished. I pressed the phone hard against my ear, waiting for some words of hope, but none came. And my world began to spin. My head felt as though it was floating away from my body. No one had died. No one was going to die today, and yet I felt like an essential part of me was dying.

I can assure you that no one ever wants to see an MRI report like I received, and I still feel a little sick to my stomach reading it: defects, delamination, tears, early degenerative changes, fraying, edema, and fat necrosis—to name but a few of the words that jumped out at me.

Thus began what turned out to be six months (the injury kept me from running for a total of 10 months) of battling depression, feeling futile, and desperately searching for some hope. At 44 years old, with a 15-month-old daughter, I was in constant pain. I would look at my daughter and cry, knowing I would never be able to go for a hike with her, frustrated because the pain made me cranky and short-tempered. Every morning as the sun streamed through our bedroom windows and beckoned me to run and run and run, I would curl up in a ball and sob.

My husband was incredulous. "Don't believe it. Don't give up," he argued. I vacillated, one moment denying the very possibility of the diagnosis—after all, I *never* had knee pain, ever—and then just as quickly the pendulum would swing, and I berated myself for succumbing to denial of the facts—the *facts*. The MRI was fact. That my knee never hurt, that this made no sense—those facts sank to the bottom of my morose soul.

Importantly, not a single doctor examined me. Not once. They told me I was done based on the imaging and my age. That was it. Nothing could be done. Case closed. But something in me didn't give up. I took my little MRI DVD down to Steadman and Hawkins in Denver. As I sat on the examination table, the doctor walked in and instantly said, "Your knee is fine. You have tendinitis." I cannot even begin to explain what those words meant to me.

Of course, it still hadn't gotten better two months later, so I visited Steadman and Hawkins again, this time asking the questions I should have asked two months prior.

Me: "So. When you told me what I wanted to hear, I forgot to ask any questions. I just wanted to go home and run again. But I still can't run, and it still isn't better, so I guess I need to ask you to explain why the MRI is wrong."

Doc: "Let me tell you a story: I have a sore back. My wife keeps telling me to get an MRI. I keep telling her I don't want to know what's going on in there. After 35, we all have arthritis, bulging discs, and other changes that may not be symptomatic. You now know things that might be better left unknown, but those are asymptomatic. Your problem now is tendinitis. Will you ever need a knee replacement? I can't answer that."

I left the office both hopeful and anxious, thinking, "I need this fixed, and I need to do the things I've been putting off for later *now*, or I may never be able to do them." And yet, in the back of my mind hung this lingering concern: What if he were wrong?

It wasn't very easy to fix, but I didn't give up and managed to stumble onto something that helped: dry needling. Over the course of two months of needling twice a week, I was running again. It was just a little bit, but I was grateful and hopeful for the first time in many months.

I adopted the attitude that I need to do what I want to do *now*. I have now. I may not have later. I already knew deep down that all I have is now, but that idea was pressed upon me more forcefully when I thought I'd lost it all. Yes, this was not a life-threatening situation (though I have since had one of those as well), and it is only running, but running matters to me, and I can't take tomorrow for granted.

> I'll be happy if running and I can grow old together.
>
> *Haruki Murakami*

Since my running days were proclaimed to be over a little more than 10 years ago, I have run over 60 races that were between marathon and 100-mile distances. I have run Boston six times, New York three times (as a time qualifier), Chicago a couple times, and various trail races all over the country. For the past seven years, I've been trying to get into the Western States Endurance Run, which requires yearly qualifiers in specific 100K or 100-mile races. I have run thousands and thousands of miles all over the world, exploring places I never would have seen otherwise and learning about myself in ways I never would have fathomed 10 years ago. And I am nowhere near done.

ACKNOWLEDGMENTS

> Man often becomes what he believes himself to be. If I keep on saying to myself that I cannot do a certain thing, it is possible that I may end by really becoming incapable of doing it. On the contrary, if I have the belief that I can do it, I shall surely acquire the capacity to do it even if I may not have it at the beginning.
>
> *Mahatma Gandhi*

Several years ago, I left my career in teaching college and dove headfirst into coaching. That necessitated a significant overhaul in my education and skill set, diving back into education as a student again—and a student I will remain always as I continue to learn and grow as a coach. But coaching is also teaching, and I still see myself first as a teacher. What I find in coaching are eager students who want to hear what I have to offer. This book is an extension of my desire to teach and guide—only on a larger scale.

I want to start by thanking all the athletes I've had the privilege to work with over the years: for trusting me, listening to me, and collaborating with me—because this is always a team effort. Thank you for providing me with the learning experiences and opportunities I could not have had any other way. Coaching is an art and an empirical practice, and you've provided me the opportunity to develop my skills, my understanding of the practical application of principles, and my knowledge.

I cannot say enough about how grateful I am to have support and encouragement from my family: My husband, Peter Beal, and my daughter, Sophia Beal-MacMahon, endured many months of my stress over struggling with writer's block, meeting deadlines, balancing demanding commitments, and just wondering if I could really finish this project. Writing a book is so much more than *just* writing, and their encouragement and belief in me kept me going, even when I doubted myself.

To Michelle Earle and Laura Pulliam at Human Kinetics: There is no way I could have completed this project without your guidance, patience, and steady, positive pressure. Your constructive feedback and attention to detail were essential for this first-time author. You both trusted me, guided me, and reassured me, which spurred me on.

Thank you to all the teachers and mentors who have guided me throughout my life, who believed in me, and who set an example of what it is to teach and encourage with integrity while living a meaningful life, including my mentor at Wells College, Laura Purdy, the first person who really entertained my questions and encouraged me to ask more; my advisor at University of Southern Maine, William Gavin, who pressed me on to graduate school because he saw something in me that was different; and my mentor and advisor at University of Colorado–Boulder, Claudia Mills, who showed me that balancing competing passions in life is hard but doable. And then there are all my USA Track and Field/World Athletics teachers and colleagues: Terry Crawford, who gave me her encouraging tough love; Joe Vigil; Jack Daniels; Gunter Lange; Robert Chapman; Scott Christensen; and so many more who have shared their knowledge and experience with me.

Finally, I want to thank, and remember, my dear friend and chiropractor—and the person who was always there when I needed to be fixed—over the past 17 years, Marc Cahn. Marc died in a tragic accident in Hawaii in March 2024. He was a serious cyclist and Deadhead, but he is also the only reason that I am still running today after being told in 2008 that my running days were over. We all need a team behind us—whether you are an elite runner or you are the last runner crossing the finish or you just want to enjoy your constitutional trot each day, you need others to guide and help you. Marc was my go-to when any little body issue showed up. I miss him immensely every day. And I was blessed to have found him when I did. Thank you, Marc.

And to you, the reader, I am profoundly grateful to you for picking up this book and joining me on this long running journey.

PART I

RUNNING

Chapter 1

Run by Your Own Rules: Understanding Realities Are Not Restrictions

> It is a shame for a man to grow old without seeing the beauty
> and strength of which his body is capable.
>
> *Socrates*

There's a quip that has become popular over the past 10 years or so: "50 is the new 30." I remember it became a common saying around the time I turned 50, so of course I found it very appealing. But is this true? Can a 50-year-old train like a 30-year-old? Can a 60- or 70-year-old train like a 30- or 40-year-old? Well, truth be told, we are still learning about this. While we understand some of the expected normal physical changes that everyone must face as they age, what we are seeing, empirically, is that older athletes keep pushing the boundaries of what they believe, or believed, to be possible. This does not just concern physical realities; it also concerns mental, emotional, spiritual, and social expectations and horizons.

The idea, reinforced by Western culture, that aging is nothing but a slow slide into inevitable decline is just not true. And while there are certainly some outliers whose lifestyles seem able to defy the effects of aging, most of you are capable of far more than you think. But you must believe and have goals and dreams that are wildly audacious and yet reachable. I always tell my athletes, "If it doesn't scare you just a little bit, consider a bigger goal." One of the most appealing aspects of running is that it provides an opportunity for each of you to choose your own adventure of sorts. Your goals may change based on what you've done in the past, when you started running, and what you truly enjoy pursuing. There really is no limit to creativity in running.

In this chapter, we'll explore the physical, mental, and social impacts of running and aging and how your relationship to running, whether this is a new relationship or one you've been in for years, will change and develop in a multitude of ways. No relationship continues without change. While we'll look more specifically at these changes with each chapter, it is important to understand that sometimes the decline of one ability comes with the improvement of another.

> Man . . . sacrifices his health in order to make money.
> Then he sacrifices money to recuperate his health.
> And then he is so anxious about the future that he does not
> enjoy the present; the result being that he does not live
> in the present or the future; he lives as if he is never going to die,
> and then dies having never really lived.
>
> *The Dalai Lama on what surprises him most about humanity*

Physical, Mental, Social, and Spiritual Factors

When running races, I see all kinds of signs held up by cheering spectators. My favorite is this: "One day you won't be able to do this. Today is not that day." I first saw this one while running my first 50-miler at the age of 51. It got me thinking for quite a few miles. Every time I run, I embrace the truth as it is in that moment—which is that I actually can do this *now*. Will there come a time when I can no longer do it? I can't possibly know that. All I can do is live my life like it matters *now*, and that means continuing to do the things I can while taking care of my body, mind, and spirit so I can keep at it for as long as my desire takes me.

So, why does running matter so much to me and, I believe, to so many others? If you're reading this book, there must be something about running that matters deeply to you. Running is just about the simplest activity possible, and yet it seems to connect you to a part of yourself that allows you to feel more alive. I'm going to take a chance here and tell you a little story or two—or rather, give you my philosophical view on running and human nature and what it is to live a good life. The fact is that you're alive, but are you really living?

Story number one: I came to coach running as both a teacher and a lifelong runner. For many years, I taught college philosophy, something that you tend to apply to your own life experiences. My area of specialty is ethics and social and political philosophy. Many years ago, I wrote a paper on eudaemonia—Aristotle's view of a flourishing life or a life well lived as a human being. According to Aristotle, everything has a "distinctive excellence" or telos, the thing it does better than anything else. A table is a table because it functions as a table better than anything else functions as a table. You may use a chair as a table, but it doesn't function as a table very well. It does, as I like to say, "chairness" better. What something does better than anything else makes a thing what it is. And its *good* is doing that thing excellently.

Let's take a table with one short leg. It still functions as a table, but it's not functioning well. It is not an excellent table. Likewise, a hand is a hand when it can function as a hand. It holds things, manipulates things, and does other hand things. Now let's cut the hand off. There lies the hand on the floor. It can no longer do hand things, though it still looks like a hand. In this case, Aristotle would say, it is a hand in name only; it is no longer actually a hand.

Now, for humans, Aristotle asks, what do we do better than anything else? He explores some obvious options, such as biological growth. But that can't be it. After all, even viruses do that, and arguably better than humans do. After many considerations, he came to a conclusion: We are moral, social, and political beings. That's what makes you human. When you are functioning well, you achieve eudaemonia, simplistically translated as "happiness" but meant more robustly as flourishing, living a good or excellent human life. I won't debate whether Aristotle got this right. I'm telling you this for one reason, and it's that I believe Aristotle missed one piece, and that is—you guessed it—running. In particular, distance running.

Why would I add something so silly and seemingly superficial to something as important as "distinctive excellence"? Well, humans do running, at least running long distances, very well. And while researchers want to argue over whether we are or are not the best at it—due to our highly developed calf muscles, ability to efficiently dissipate heat through sweat, upright posture that limits sun exposure, and short toes—the truth remains that sometimes we run just to run. We can look to all the evolutionary stories, but none explains why we *like* to run.

Arguably, endurance running is something we do very well, but it is also something that may also allow us to flourish emotionally, mentally, spiritually, socially, and physically. Sometimes we go out for a run just because we want to—not to get somewhere or win something or catch anything but just to run. In these cases, we run as an end in itself, not for something else. Do other animals do this? I have no idea. I often see horses and cows run and frolic in the fields, sometimes racing around, but do they set off to run for 10 or 100 miles just because they feel like it?

Moreover, Aristotle asserts that happiness requires exertion, meaning action. Happiness is not passive. If my theory holds and running is part of a flourishing human life, then this does not change as you grow older, though it may become more challenging to pursue. But eudaemonia is not something you achieve and then you're done. It's a continual process of being until you are no longer being.

Story number two: John Stuart Mill, the father of liberalism and utilitarian ethics, presented compelling moral and political philosophies, but his concerns were very pragmatic and empirical: His aim was to figure out how to maximize happiness for the greatest number. He wanted more happiness in the world. But what is happiness? What he suggested is that humans who function generally well are happiest when they enjoy the higher pleasures. Lower pleasures are easy to enjoy but add little to your sense of self-mastery or self-worth. Higher pleasures are those that do not come easily but add to your sense of self. They challenge you, and when you rise to the occasion, you come to understand your abilities and your power.

Let's consider two pleasures: watching a football game versus playing a football game. Mill would argue that you get a deeper satisfaction from playing the game (challenging) than from watching the game (easy). Difficult things make you feel better about yourself, and that leads to a more robust type of happiness. It's not that you cannot enjoy simple, lower pleasures, but you cannot *only* enjoy those, because the functionality of your being demands more. Like Aristotle's, Mill's idea of happiness requires exertion and effort. It is not passive. Add to this the claim that more units of happiness—each person counts as a unit—create more happiness in the world, resulting in a better world, and it's clear that activities like running contribute to both our happiness and the greater good.

You are not meant to be a spectator in life. You are meant to live, really live, for as many years as you have. Humans seem to be happiest when taking on a challenge, whatever it may be. This never ends until you take your last breath, and maybe not even then. The great thing about running is that there are so many options. I call running the choose-your-own-adventure part of life. For many of you, running is more than an activity you do; it's part of who you are.

Allow me to tie this all together by considering the arguments of yet another philosopher. William James argued three important points that I believe apply here:

1. You create your reality through your beliefs.
2. You are morally permitted to make choices about things you may never have absolute knowledge about.
3. When you truly believe something, you act on it. If you say you believe something but your actions don't reflect that belief, then you don't actually believe it.

When I taught college philosophy, I used to demonstrate this first point with the following story: Sometime in the 1990s—I don't remember exactly when—a radio DJ in Denver pulled a prank on listeners, claiming that someone had set hundreds of chickens free in the city and that they were frantically running through the streets. As a result, listeners started racing around the city looking for these poor, hapless chickens to save them from certain death on the city streets. Now, in reality there were no chickens, but if you looked at the actions of the people rushing around, you would see a situation where many people were clearly looking for something. And if you asked them what they were looking for, they would tell you, "We're looking for the loose chickens." They believed it, and their actions reflected that belief, so in effect, they created the truth through those actions.

James' second point concerns important beliefs you hold about claims you can't have absolute certainty about. Let's take love as an example: Can you *know* with certainty that someone loves you? Well, you can ask them, and they may tell you they do, but does that mean you *know* they do? They either do or they do not, and it's uncertain whether you know the truth. But there is an answer. There is truth. In this case, you have the right to choose to believe that they love you. You may be wrong, or you may be right. You are not required to wait for more evidence to present itself. Unlike matters of science, sometimes you are faced with questions and decisions that cannot be decided on purely intellectual ground. These concern passionate beliefs—whom you love, how you live your life—and they cannot be avoided. You may never have proof that someone loves you or that you chose the right sort of life to live, but you can't sit around waiting for an absolute answer. Making a choice to live a certain way changes your life.

When you truly believe something, you act on it. If the belief doesn't lead to action, then your belief amounts to nothing but empty, meaningless words. If, for example, I believe that eating a healthy diet will make me feel better, but I continue to eat junk, then I don't really believe what I say I believe.

> Act as if what you do makes a difference. It does.
>
> *William James*

Combine all of this and you have a compelling argument for the value of living a vibrant and active life for your body, mind, and spirit. And this leads to my next consideration. A recent development in running is the considerable increase in the number of new runners 50 or over entering the sport (Marcus 2023). There are so many new runners lacing up their running shoes and hitting the roads and trails. Perhaps they have been involved in other sports all along, or perhaps they are returning to activity after a long layoff. It's quite common to see former high school or college runners return to the sport in their 50s and 60s because many adult responsibilities, including working demanding jobs and raising families, take priority in your 20s, 30s, and 40s. For these folks, a little slack in demands allows them to think about getting back to something they may have been missing a bit all these years.

There are also the newer runners who may have never been involved in any sport but somehow find their way to running later in life. I see many reasons offered for this new discovery: physical and mental health issues, weight concerns, trouble quitting drinking or smoking, desire for a healthier lifestyle, exploration of the world around them, social interaction through running groups and races, personal journeys, rehabilitation from an illness or injury, peer pressure, involvement in their kids' sports, midlife crisis, loss of a spouse or partner, divorce, and the list goes on and on. Many feel the march of time; they see the effects on those around them, and they wish to improve their health and habits.

There are also the runners who have been running for years and have just kept running. I've been running most of my life, and like many other longtime runners, it's simply part of who I am. It's just what I do. When I was racing as a young adult, older runners were a rarity. I remember one man in my running club in Maine who was in his 70s at the time. As a 25-year-old, I admired his enthusiasm, energy, and wisdom, and I hoped to be like him when I got older. These outliers set an example for me, and now I'm seeing the results of that. Some of you no longer believe you must give up an active life just because you reach a certain age. And today you have even more examples of athletes over 50 crushing previously held misconceptions. In turn, you are creating new possibilities for those who follow you.

> The obsession with running is really an obsession with the potential for more and more life.
>
> *George Sheehan*

Societal Expectations

As you get older, you face new challenges. But are these challenges real or imagined? Are they deal killers, or are there things you can do to help your changing situation? Continuing to run, to pursue goals whatever those may be, or beginning to run, maybe for the first time, requires courage. It requires you to do things others may believe are unwise or even foolhardy.

> A man with outward courage dares to die;
> a man with inner courage dares to live.
>
> *Lao Tzu*

The issues facing older athletes are not just physical in nature; significant social conditioning and expectations figure into the equation. Your concept of yourself is highly influenced by societal expectations. Most people view older athletes as weaker, slower, and generally declining. This is not something you look forward to, but it's often something you are told to expect, accept, and deal with. As you get older, you are discouraged from engaging in physical activity that is too intense, too vigorous, or too stressful. You're told that you need to worry about your knees or your heart. Why? Because exercise is often seen as pointless and dangerous for older people. Why would you run a race if you weren't trying to win it? Why would you run if you weren't getting any faster and might even get slower? This is the winner-takes-all mentality that causes many people to stop doing so many things they care deeply about.

You may run a race, and that race may be very important to you even though you have no chance of winning. Or maybe you're competing against other people your age, and that matters to you. Maybe you're competing against yourself. Maybe you're tackling something completely new, something you're not sure you can complete. Maybe your goal is to run a new route through your neighborhood or make it up that hill without walking. Maybe you want to run because you enjoy being outside, moving through the world, experiencing the changing of seasons, and letting your thoughts flow. Maybe you run because it allows you to feel strong and healthy. As Woody Allen famously said, "Eighty percent of success in life is showing up." Whether it's for the sake of physical and mental health, something you just enjoy doing, a competitive drive, or simply a means to explore your abilities and limitations—whatever the reason, keep showing up and see what happens. Stop showing up, and the die is cast.

Society as a whole is conflicted about growing older. Some well-intentioned family members, friends, and doctors will say that age is just a number while also urging you to watch how much you do. On the one hand, there are those who say, "All I need to do is keep running, and when I'm 50 I'll be able to qualify for Boston." Clearly the 20- and 30-somethings see the qualifying times for older folks as easily attainable. On the other hand, some older runners and mostly nonrunners I know begin to believe they can't really run or push themselves the way they wish they could—or at all—and sometimes use their age as an excuse to not even try. Now, if they just don't want to, that's fine, but let's stop using age as an excuse. Age itself is not a disability or a disease. In many cultures, age is respected and revered. In ours, it is pitied and dreaded. While age is certainly more than just a number, it's not something that seals you into a fate of regretful decline. You can look at the challenges of aging and adapt. But first you must shake some of the preconceptions you have absorbed over the years.

If you focus a lot more on what older people continue to accomplish and less on the culture of youth, you'll contribute to a happier, healthier, more vibrant society as a whole. There are strengths older athletes may possess, and those can be capitalized upon.

I believe that a lot of people feel old because they're told they are old and should feel old. For years and years, even my own mother asked me when I was going to slow down on the running thing. At this point, she's given up asking, and though she's not a runner, she still exercises twice a day at the age of 85—even as a cancer survivor and kidney failure survivor and with various other mortal threats breathing down her neck.

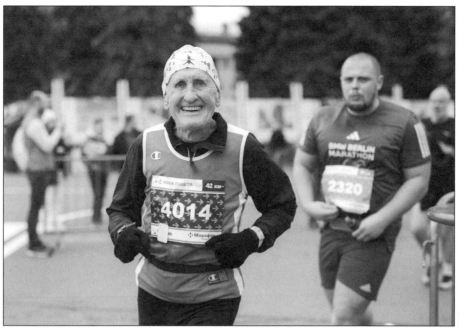

Of course, aging is not just a social construct. There are physiological things going on that need to be taken into account and individual variabilities to acknowledge. Genetics and life circumstances, both in and out of your control, affect these things. But to simply stop doing the things that bring value to your life just because you're 50 or 60 or 70 is shortsighted and sad. Life has the depth and breadth that you bring to it. A full life can last a full lifetime. I still have many audacious goals I yearn to pursue. Perhaps some people look at me as someone deep in denial. But as William James argued, in terms of your lived experience, you create your reality through your beliefs.

> Human beings, by changing the inner attitudes of their minds, can change the outer aspects of their lives.
>
> *William James*

Physical Changes

Recently, another runner over 50 mentioned to me that his doctor informed him he should have stopped running after he turned 50. I asked why? Apparently his doctor did not attempt to justify his prescription for inactivity. He simply said it was too much stress. A couple years ago when I was probably 55, shortly after finishing my fourth 100-miler, I went in for a routine physical. When I told my doctor what I had been up to, she looked at me and said, "You know you can't do these things forever." While that's an obvious truth, I have yet to find a doctor who knows when doing these things will no longer be feasible. Until I find them, I will keep doing what I can do.

You hear time and again from medical professionals that running will wear you out, that you need to back off, slow down, and accept the realities of aging. But—and this is important—just because you refuse to give in doesn't mean that there are no real challenges to deal with. While you do create your reality in many meaningful ways, you must also deal with physical realities that are not entirely yours to control. But the overwhelming evidence, even given the inevitability of aging and some decline, is that running statistically delays the effects of aging. Mobility, balance, flexibility, muscle strength and recruitment, cardiac and lung function, speed and efficiency, and mental acuity and mental health all benefit from running. Even cognitive decline is reduced with consistent exercise.

One truth that exists for all bodies, young or old, is that the body is efficient. The body will not maintain what it does not need. Why would the body maintain heavy, energy-intensive bones and muscles if they weren't needed? This is absolutely the use-it-or-lose-it principle. You do not build strength in any bodily structure and then just rely on it to be there for the duration of your life. So if you have weak ankles, for example, should you wear a brace or do ankle-strengthening exercises? Unless you want even weaker ankles, you better toss the brace and embrace the strength training. Now, obviously there are times to brace and support bodily structures, specifically when they are healing from an injury, but if you are adding support because something feels weak, that will only serve to further weaken the already frail structure.

So the real issue is what physical reality entails and what you can do to give yourself the best possible chances in life. There are some general changes, or possible changes, and physiological factors to keep in mind.

Recovery Time

For all athletes—and everyone out there moving their bodies is an athlete, no matter what level—recovery time matters. Some athletes notice that as time marches on, they need more time to recover. Perhaps you can no longer do hard runs day after day, or you find that you need to cut mileage or that speed or hill workouts don't work well every week. Training will change over time. It doesn't matter what your age is—if you keep doing the same thing over and over, you will never progress. Recovery has always been important for real improvement, but as is the case for many things, younger runners can get away with bad training for a longer time than older runners. That doesn't mean it's good for them to neglect recovery, but they may not feel the effects as quickly or dramatically.

Many see recovery as separate from training, but recovery *is* training. Improvement happens when you stress your system and then allow your body to absorb and adapt to the training through recovery. Stress plus recovery equals increased strength. Training is the whole system: the hard days, the easy days, the rest days, and the cross-training days. Recovery weeks are crucial for athletes of any age. Those should come every three to four weeks.

Also, sleep is more important than ever. Generally, human growth hormone (HGH) also decreases as you age, but when you sleep, your HGH does its job and reaches its peak. What that means for athletes over 50 is that sleep is one of the most important recovery tools in your tool belt. In addition to sleep, nutrition is an often neglected factor in being able to recover well. Postrun nutrition must be priority one, and overall general nutrition needs serious attention. Protein becomes more important as you age. With intense speed and strength work, protein encourages stronger muscles and connective tissues. To maximize postrun recovery, nutrition is a priority, and nutrients should ideally be consumed within 20 minutes of finishing your workout. This also restocks your muscle glycogen for your next workout.

Muscle Mass

Muscle mass slowly decreases over time. Involuntary loss of muscle mass is referred to as *sarcopenia* and often contributes to disability in older people. Sarcopenia begins as early as your 40s and continues linearly until your 80s. The reasons for this are still very much in dispute, but it appears there may be many factors, including metabolic and endocrine changes. The number one risk factor leading to decreased muscle mass and disability is inactivity. One problem, however, is that there are no standardized measurements to determine and track muscle loss because experts disagree on the definition of sarcopenia.

However, age-related muscle loss can be prevented and even reversed with exercise. This is good news whether your aim is to run for health, competition, enjoyment of the outdoors, or whatever your why is. Furthermore, aerobic activity improves your maximal oxygen consumption ($\dot{V}O_2$max), increases your mitochondrial density and size (your ATP factories), and boosts your protein synthesis, insulin sensitivity, and neuromuscular function. While aerobic activity alone may not lead to noticeable muscle hypertrophy, it does enhance muscle strength, quality, and function.

Add in resistance and strength training. When running, add some fast strides—short, controlled accelerations, not sprints—at the end of a couple runs a week. Or do a fartlek once or twice a week. *Fartlek* is Swedish for "speed play," and it can actually be fun. You can take a run and turn it into a game; press the uphills or downhills, or speed up for every turn or when a car passes. Race to that next tree or rock or lamppost—make it fun. Or you can add in a hilly route once a week, but now push the uphills harder. There are so many options. Intensity doesn't require you to go to a track and run 400-meter repeats until you feel like you could puke.

Joint Health

Articular cartilage, which lines the bones in your joints, tends to thin over time. Ligaments and tendons also lose elasticity. As a result, joints can feel tight and painful. But running and other activity helps maintain joint health. Contrary to common opinion, knees do not wear out. Over time, you will not ruin your knees from running. This has been shown in study after study (Alentorn-Geli et al. 2017). In fact, there appears to be an inverse relationship. Those who have a history of running tend to have less knee pain over their lifetime (Lo et al. 2017). When you run or walk, the movement increases synovial fluid in the joint capsule. Synovial fluid is to the knee what motor oil is to an engine—it lubricates the joint and keeps things running smoothly. Movement also keeps ligaments and tendons more pliable because it increases circulation, which is crucial for ligament and tendon health.

Bone Health

Many see bones as unchanging tissues. They develop when you're young, and then they're just there for the duration of your life—homeostasis. But this is probably not the case. It doesn't matter if you're 25 or 55; bones are dynamic and ever-changing based on the stress they must adapt to. The use-it-or-lose-it adage applies to bones as much as to any other part of the body. You are led to believe that all you need to do is get enough calcium and your bones will stay strong and healthy. However, that may not actually be how things work.

Wolff's law, formulated by the German anatomist Julius Wolff in the 19th century, is a principle that describes how bone adapts to mechanical stress over time. When bones are subjected to stress or load, such as through weight-bearing exercise or physical activity, they grow stronger and denser to better withstand those forces. But in areas where there is reduced stress or load, bones weaken and lose density.

Importantly, Wolff's law does not really address the nutrition side of things or the actual mechanism of stress, which is important to add to the picture. The Utah paradigm builds on Wolff's law. The Utah paradigm emphasizes the importance of mechanical loading for bone health. It suggests that bones respond to mechanical stress by undergoing a process called remodeling, which involves the removal of old or damaged bone tissue (resorption via osteoclasts) followed by the formation of new bone tissue (formation via osteoblasts). This continuous remodeling process helps bones adapt to changing mechanical demands, such as weight-bearing activities or resistance training. It turns out that the only way to make and keep a bone strong is by exerting force on the bone. Let's take a look at a few things that factor into healthy bones:

- *Nutrition:* Adequate intake of essential nutrients, particularly calcium and vitamin D, is crucial for bone health. Calcium is a key mineral component of bones, while vitamin D aids in calcium absorption. Other nutrients such as magnesium, phosphorus, and vitamin K are also important for bone metabolism.
- *Weight-bearing exercise:* Weight-bearing exercises, such as walking, running, jumping, and resistance training, stimulate bone remodeling and promote bone formation. These activities subject bones to mechanical stress, triggering them to become stronger and denser over time.
- *Hormonal balance:* Hormones play a significant role in bone metabolism. Estrogen, testosterone, and HGH are among the hormones that influence bone health. Maintaining hormonal balance through your lifestyle and, if necessary, medical interventions can support bone building and reduce the risk of bone loss.
- *Mineralization:* Ensuring sufficient mineralization of the bone matrix is essential for bone strength. This involves maintaining proper levels of minerals such as calcium, phosphorus, and magnesium as well as promoting the deposition of these minerals into the bone matrix.
- *Prevention of bone loss:* Strategies to prevent bone loss are integral to the Utah paradigm. This includes avoiding factors that contribute to bone loss, such as smoking, excessive alcohol consumption, and certain medications, as well as addressing underlying medical conditions that may affect bone health (Frost 2000).

Researchers are still arguing about the actual mechanisms and roles of both mechanical and nonmechanical influences. But the takeaway is this: The body does not waste energy maintaining unnecessary structures. Dense bones can be heavy and require a lot of bodily resources to build and maintain. If you need those dense bones, based on the demands you make on them, then your body will produce the resources necessary to maintain them, assuming you have the nutrients available. And when you aren't providing those nutrients, the body will find them if it can, which is why a pregnant woman's body will take minerals from her bones to support the growing baby if she isn't supplying enough. But it's the physical demands that initiate the response. The force that muscles, tendons, and ligaments put on bones gets the nutrients where they need to be. Without strong muscles, you will not have strong bones.

Are Runners Over 50 More Prone to Injury?

The answer is maybe, maybe not. A lot depends on how recovery is balanced with training—and life—stresses. As you age, your bones tend to get smaller and less dense. Why? It's believed that as you get older, you absorb less calcium and vitamin D, which are crucial to bone health. But the Utah paradigm and Wolff's law suggest that it is not just calcium and vitamin D at issue—what matters even before all that is the stress on the bone. What kind of stress? Specifically, it is the stress caused by muscles pulling on opposite ends of the bone. Impact is one thing, but it's the actual pull of the muscle on the bone that provides the stimulus for calcium uptake. You can consume all the calcium in the world and still have weak bones if you do not stress them. Without the stress, calcium will not go into your bones. Period.

Cardiac Output

Blood vessels and arteries lose their elasticity as you age. This means they are less able to expand when blood is being pumped through them, potentially leading to higher blood pressure and reduced max heart rate. While older hearts may function well, that function decreases when maximum effort is made. The heart just doesn't pump as fast or pump as much volume as a younger heart. The good news is that regular aerobic activity slows this process and improves heart function. Remember, the heart is a muscle. It needs to be worked to stay strong. Also note that as your maximum heart rate goes down, so does your $\dot{V}O_2$max. But training can cut this decline in half. Your $\dot{V}O_2$max indicates how efficiently and effectively you can take oxygen into your lungs and how well your blood carries oxygen to your muscles to fuel muscle contraction.

There is a strong correlation between sedentary middle age and reduced cardiac function, which increases linearly as you age and can eventually lead to heart failure due to decreased cardiac muscle plasticity. Basically, this means that when you don't exercise through middle age, the left ventricle (LV), the part of your heart that pumps oxygen-rich blood back to your body, becomes stiff. With each pump of your heart, the LV pushes less and less blood back into the body. Research strongly suggests that exercise, even if you've been sedentary, can reverse this through middle age. Those who engage in moderately intense exercise maintain the LV function of much younger individuals. However, it's important to note, at least with previously sedentary people, intensity and duration matters, and the prescription for improved cardiac function is a bit higher than for a general exercise prescription. You don't need to be a high-level competitive masters runner, but you do need to include some more intense running. Additionally, those who have been running through middle age or earlier (i.e., they have not been sedentary leading up to middle age) show cardiac function similar to younger populations.

The takeaway here is this: If you are 45 to 64 years old and sedentary, you still have a chance to reverse this decline in cardiac function due to LV stiffening. After 65, this response to exercise decreases exponentially, to the point where current research shows no improvement for sedentary individuals. That does not mean it's too late to start, even if you're 65 or older, but that improvements in this area are smaller. It's clear that sedentary aging leads to cardiac stiffness, which at some point is irreversible (Howden et al. 2018).

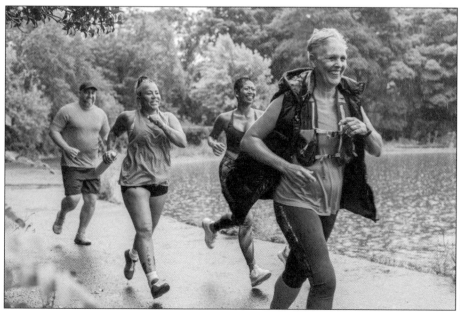

Body Composition

A recent and very compelling study suggests that, contrary to anecdotal tales of woefully inevitable weight gain, your metabolism may not come to a screeching halt on your 50th birthday (Pontzer et al. 2021). In fact, this study found that metabolism begins to slow at a steady rate from about age 30 until 60. At 60, things pick up a bit, but not to the extent that it explains the ever-expanding girth of the average middle-aged and older American—and others around the globe who have adopted an American lifestyle. This story isn't just about metabolism; it's also about changes in muscles, hormones (something we'll discuss later), and diet.

Flexibility and Mobility

Functional mobility means you can comfortably move your joints through all planes of motion, requiring not just healthy joints but healthy connective tissue to support and move those joints. If you do dynamic drills that move your body through all the planes, use free weights to work all the muscles, tendons, and ligaments used to stabilize your joints, and weave in activities like yoga or swimming, you will keep up your ability to run, twist, jump, and skip. Staying active is crucial to maintain mobility because movement increases the synovial fluid in your joints, which makes movement easier. When you aren't active, you slide into a vicious circle: Inactivity leads to feeling stiff, which reduces movement, which progresses to pain, which then results in even less movement. You have to keep moving in order to keep moving. And once you stop moving, it's not just your muscles and connective tissues that deteriorate; your entire body begins to break down. Mentally, it can be hard to be in pain, unable to do the basic things you want to do. Socially, becoming inactive can be isolating.

Running form, which has been a focus of attention for the past 10 years or so, is also something that will benefit from improved flexibility and mobility. Dynamic warm-up drills help set you up for more efficient movement. If you're concerned about slowing down, look at the two main elements of speed: stride length (the amount of ground you cover per step) and cadence (the number of steps you take per minute). Generally, your stride length shortens and your foot turnover slows as you age. Working on your flexibility and mobility can improve both. It can also improve how you carry yourself when running.

Hormonal Changes

As you get older, the anabolic hormones testosterone and estrogen begin to decrease. What that means is that you must work hard to make the most of what you have. Adding intensity and strength work uses those hormones to their best advantage. HGH also decreases, which makes recovery more difficult. HGH does its most important work during sleep. You'll learn more about HGH later in chapter 7. As I tell my coached athletes, sleep is the number one recovery tool. Quantity and quality both matter.

To sum up, the key to addressing all these changes is to train smart, take recovery seriously, and eat well—that doesn't mean you have to be perfect. While you do slow a bit over time, it's actually not that dramatic, and you can do a lot to slow down the decline. But best of all, continuing to run will allow you to maintain your quality of life. And that's really what it's all about: living a long, rich life.

While 50 may not entirely be the new 30, age brings with it both new challenges and new strengths. In life, you are always presented with a menu of choices, and those options change over time. It is important to know that, barring particular individual limitations, you can continue to pursue a physically active life that will confer physical, mental, and social benefits, allowing you to remain vibrant throughout your life.

Chapter 2

Find Your Drive: Determining Goals and Creating Habits

Some seasoned runners continue to pursue lofty goals—faster times or longer races. Do you still want to beat your 10K personal record (PR) from when you were 25? Is it possible to top those 20-something times? Or maybe over the years you've pursued different goals. Maybe you've been running marathons and want to try an ultramarathon. Perhaps you've never been a runner but want to start. Is it too late?

Well, a lot depends on how you were training then and how you're training now. It's certainly more difficult as you get older, but it's not out of the question. For elite runners who trained optimally and ran world bests in their 20s and 30s, the likelihood of continuing to run those fast times into their 50s and beyond is unlikely. But for most non-elite athletes, continuing to run close to your personal bests may be more feasible with smart and efficient training. It's certainly easier to get away with poor training and suboptimal choices and still pull off impressive times when you're younger. But as with most things, as you get older, you need to work smarter. When the margin for error decreases, you start to feel the real effects of poor habits and inappropriate goals.

Training Smarter

I've seen many runners 50 and over continuing to do what they've always done, and when that stops working, they often feel frustrated and believe the solution lies in doing more—more miles, more speed work, more of something. But more may not be the solution.

Let's take Joanna, a 55-year-old who is training for a marathon: She's experienced and has trained through many marathon cycles, but this time she feels like she's working harder even though her paces keep dropping. In frustration, she tries to run more and faster. She begins feeling deep fatigue and watches as her easy pace becomes more and more difficult to run. As she continues to push harder and harder, she basically digs herself into a deeper and deeper hole: Her times slow, her fatigue increases, her body begins to hurt, her heart rate both at rest and when active rises, she feels irritable, her sleep is a mess, she can't seem to concentrate on anything, and she feels like she'll never feel strong again. She wonders: Is this just part of getting old?

Next, we have Joe, a new runner. He's 58 and has never run. He has a few pounds to lose, but he's generally healthy and wants to stay that way. Both his parents died too young from heart disease, and he doesn't want to follow in their footsteps. He starts running two miles a day, four to five days a week. He's vexed because he can't seem to run any farther or faster, and his shins and knees are starting to hurt.

He just doesn't know what to do next. He wonders: Is it just too late to start running?

The solution for both runners is better, smarter training. Smart training begins with listening to your body. Of course, a good training plan is key, but if you aren't listening to your body, then you end up injured, exhausted, plateaued, and ready to give up in disgust. Too many people believe you need to beat your body into submission if you want to get fitter, stronger, and faster. You can thank Friedrich Nietzsche—who famously said, "That which does not kill us makes us stronger"—for encouraging this self-destructive tendency. Maybe this applies to some things, but when you approach training this way all the time, it will certainly leave you a broken mess.

So, what should you be listening to? Let's take a look:

Resting Heart Rate

To start, you should be monitoring your resting heart rate. Every runner should know what their resting heart rate generally is, within a few points. This is your heart rate when you first wake up, but it's also good to know where your heart rate typically settles when you're just sitting and relaxing. If you notice your heart rate is a bit higher for a few days, it will benefit you to take some extra recovery time. This doesn't necessarily mean complete rest, but you need to back off both volume and effort. If you catch this early, it's quite easy to resolve. But if it's been going on for a while, then you've dug your hole deeper, and it will take more time to get out.

Sleep Quality and Quantity

Notice the quality and quantity of your sleep. One of the ironies about sleep is that often your sleep becomes poor when you are the most fatigued: you have trouble falling asleep, you wake up often and can't get back to sleep, and you wake up in the morning still feeling exhausted. Sleep disturbances often arise due to deep systemic fatigue. Often, doing less helps improve your sleep. And, as explained in chapter 1, sleep is your number one recovery tool.

Persistent Aches and Pains

Notice how your muscles feel. Some runners erroneously believe they should always feel sore. Many think that if you're sore all the time, then you're getting strong. Unfortunately, that's not how this works. Yes, you will be sore after some runs or strength work. But the key to getting stronger is allowing your body the chance to repair following a stress. If you're always sore, that's your body saying you are doing too much of something.

Slowing Paces

If you're running at the same effort but your paces are inexplicably slowing, that's your body telling you that you're doing something wrong. Most runners run just a little too fast too often. This leads to frustrating plateaus and chronic overuse injuries.

As you get older, you need to be even more attentive to your body. You also need to be more vigilant about self-care, both physical and mental. Adding gentle mobility work, restorative bodywork such as massage, purposeful cross-training, or even a good old hot bath can do the body good. The good news is, running actually helps you become more aware of what's going on with your body. You're less likely to dismiss some little ache or pain because you don't want it to interfere with your life. When I was much younger, I would try to run through anything. Sometimes I got off lucky, and other times I ran myself into a nice injury that left me sitting on the couch berating myself for my own stupidity. Today when I feel something isn't quite right, I'll take an extra easy day, go for a swim, or make an appointment for a massage. I don't want to lose time and consistency to an injury, and nipping it in the bud is by far the smartest thing to do.

With all this in mind, it's important to recognize that the key to maintaining and improving fitness is consistency. Nothing is more important to your running than consistency. This is one big reason you want to stay healthy. Injuries interrupt training. Chronic low-level pain undermines your training and, more importantly, your enjoyment. Being in pain all the time, even if you can run, just isn't fun. What *is* fun is feeling good and strong and able to do what you want to do.

Older runners may bring a mental advantage to their training and racing. Not only does physical activity help keep you mentally healthy, but as an older runner, you may have a mental advantage over your younger self. Age may not, by itself, bring mental toughness, but chances are that you have gained some mental tenacity through the trials and tribulations of life. You see in ultra-long-distance events that older runners fair very well against their younger, faster, and physically stronger competitors, often because they have the mental toughness that these grueling efforts demand.

Running also serves a social function. When you run, you're out moving through the world. Even when you're alone, you're still among others. If you run with people or in a race, you connect with an active community that supports and inspires you. Through social interaction, you become aware of all the possibilities out there, the exciting things others do, and the things you do that introduce new possibilities to others. It becomes a mutually beneficial relationship where your life expands and your expanded life helps others do the same. It's good to be around those with whom you share passions. With more older runners sticking with running and many more joining the ranks, you have even more people to share your passion with.

And while running is not the only activity that can bring these benefits, there are certain aspects inherent to running that make them easier to attain: I don't need a team. I can go at my own pace. I can choose my own goal, be that a 100-meter sprint or a 100-mile endurance run. I can run anywhere—road, trail, treadmill, even a pool. I can run on my schedule. Running is an autonomous activity.

But I believe running is more than an activity, an exercise, or a workout. Running can also help you tune into yourself, your environment, your dreams, your pain, your ambitions, your hopes. Running gives you an opportunity to discover and exercise your greatness from where you are right now.

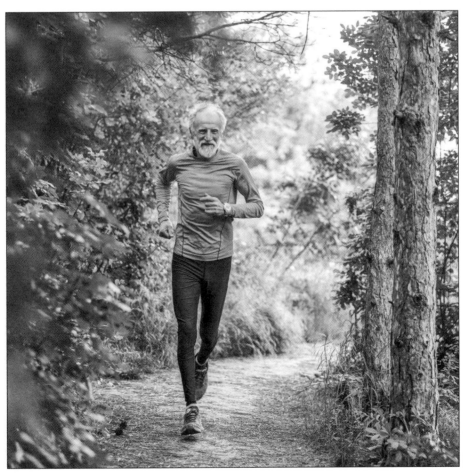

Creating Habits

There's a question I hear time and again: "How do others find the motivation to run, day in and day out?" The assumption in the question is that those who consistently run are always motivated. This is fallacious thinking, and it's what the fallacy of begging the question actually means (everyone uses that phrase wrong). The question not being asked here is, "Are those who run consistently always motivated to run?" And the assumed answer to the unstated question is yes. I could add, "And those people must have some elusive secret I want to know." I've been running steadily, consistently, day in and day out, since 1985. That's a long time, and if you think I've always been motivated, then you are sadly mistaken.

> Motivation is what gets you started.
> Habit is what keeps you going.
>
> *Jim Ryun*

Motivation is not the key here—habit is. If you wait for motivation every day, you'll never form the habit because some days you just won't want to run, and if you give in to that, then you won't run. Then every day you don't feel motivated, you stay firmly planted on the couch, and the habit you form, instead of running, is couch-sitting. Now, if that's what you're after, far be it from me to say anything about that. But these questions indicate that you don't want to develop the habit of couch-sitting; you want to run—or at least move, exercise, get out in the fresh air. But you seem to think that those who consistently run enjoy constant, unrelenting desire. When you see others out running, you wonder: How are they always so jazzed to run? This is like expecting a marriage to always be like the honeymoon or the first infatuations of love. If those are your expectations, your marriage is not going to last.

Ultimately, it comes down to what you actually want. Not what you *say* you want, but what you *really* want. The reason you sometimes fail to do what you say you want to do is that you don't really want to do it. You may say you do, but if you're not willing to do what needs to be done to achieve it, your actions show what you really desire. Take this common complaint: "I don't have the time." In most cases, you make time for the things you really value. The idea of "finding" time is one of the unhelpful myths you can believe in. You will never "find" time. In the end, your actions, not your words, show your values and desires.

I see this illustrated time and again in runners. Many will sign up for a big scary race. They'll be all excited and ready for anything. Note: the rush of adrenaline as you click "submit" on the race registration can be achieved by anyone. But then training kicks in. You hit patches where you just don't make it happen. You don't feel like going. You bemoan your regrettable lack of motivation and reach out for some hints, some guidance, on where it might be found. In the meantime, you sit back and wait for it to return.

I've literally had runners tell me, "I didn't want to get off the couch," or, "Football was on," or, "I just didn't have time to run my long run." "Um," I say. "Okay. But you do want to run that marathon, correct?" "Yes. I really do." They swear up, down, and sideways.

And then week after week and month after month, things slide. This is not about motivation; it's about deep desires and habit. So, if you can't seem to get out there due to lack of motivation, perhaps it's time to look deeply into yourself and determine whether what you *say* you want is, in fact, what you *really* want. If it is, then you need to focus on habit and let the myth of motivation go. There will be days you ride an endless wave of motivation, and there will be days you drag your sorry, obstinate self out to do what you do. Do not deceive yourself into believing that others have some magic secret that you lack. If you really want to run—if you really want to be a runner—then you will run, and that will become part of who you are.

Of course, the trick is first developing the habit. Let's briefly return to Aristotle and explore how he believed you develop your "virtues": Let's say you wish to be courageous, but right now you aren't courageous. There's only one way to become courageous, and that is to act courageously. Over time, this becomes a habit, and it gets easier to be courageous. And if you don't know what it means to be courageous, if you don't know what courage looks like, you can look to examples of courageous actions and use those as a guide for your own actions. You become what you do over and over again.

> Excellence is an art won by training and habituation. We do not act rightly because we have virtue or excellence, but we rather have those because we have acted rightly. We are what we repeatedly do. Excellence, then, is not an act but a habit.
>
> *Aristotle*

But it takes time and willingness to develop a habit, which will also include breaking a habit. Habits can, of course, be "good" or "bad." In this case, you want to develop a good habit, running, while breaking a bad habit, inactivity. Studies suggest that it takes ten weeks, give or take, to form a new habit (Gardner, Lally, and Wardle 2012). But for a habit to really take hold can take many months. This can be daunting, but it should also be encouraging, because many become discouraged when a habit doesn't settle in quickly. They enthusiastically go out for a run and then another, and then a few days later they suddenly don't feel like it, and they give in to that feeling. This is one reason why you give up on these changes you want to make. Having a realistic time frame and expectations is crucial to success.

The key to setting yourself up for success is to first set small, measurable goals. If you want to start running regularly as part of a healthier lifestyle, you need to set reasonable goals based on your starting point, not based on some grand desire off in the future. Let's take the case of a sedentary 55-year-old woman, but this example applies to everyone regardless of gender or sex. It's January, the month of resolutions, and she's set a goal of running a 10K by the end of the year. She's picked out the race and is excited to start. Where does she begin? She makes a commitment to get out the door to walk for 15 minutes, maybe a few times a week. It helps if she does this at the same time every time. For her schedule, perhaps she has a cup of coffee and something light to eat and then heads out for her walk. This becomes her cue for the new habit. Each week, her walks become a bit more frequent. Then she adds on distance or time. Then she adds in intervals of jogging. Over time, exercise begins to feel like a regular part of her day. Yes, there are those days she really isn't in the mood, but she usually goes anyway. She's always happy she went even when she didn't want to go. She starts feeling stronger. She starts eating better. She's going to sleep earlier and sleeping more soundly. Her previous habit of inactivity is no longer a natural part of her day. Her consistent doing has created the habit, and now she's beginning to feel all the benefits of that new habit, which reinforces the habit. Now on the days she doesn't run, she feels as though something is missing from her day.

> I have been impressed with the urgency of doing.
> Knowing is not enough; we must apply.
> Being willing is not enough; we must do.
>
> *Leonardo da Vinci*

Determining Goals

Based on the discussion above, it seems that goals are a necessary part of consistent running. But are goals necessary? Well, the answer to that depends on what you mean by *goal*. Goals can be ends in themselves or means to further ends. If I just enjoy the act of running, then I run as an end in itself, not for any further end or goal. Does that mean I don't have goals? No. It just means that the goal is in the action—the enjoyment of running. For years, I ran for no other reason than the daily habit of it. Running was as much a part of my day as eating. I didn't run races; I didn't want to run farther or faster; I just enjoyed my time out running each day. Other goals may involve a means to an end, but they don't need to. A goal is whatever you find value in. It's about the reason you do what you do. Tapping into what matters to you, what excites you and moves you, is all that matters.

Whether you're young or old, this is the number one piece of advice when choosing goals: Start where you are now. You need to honestly assess your current fitness and then set a reasonable time frame for achieving your goals. This may mean setting some intermediate goals. If, for instance, you're currently running a 5-mile long run and about 10 miles a week overall, but you really want to run a half-marathon in a month, understanding that may be an overreach and an invite for injury will help you dial that goal back a bit. Instead, think about a half-marathon in several months, with a healthy build toward that goal.

The second most important piece of advice is this: Think about short-, medium-, and long-term goals. These apply to all ages and all experience levels. If you have big goals, it will help to set some smaller goals along the way that are reasonable and measurable. You will see your progress, and both your fitness and your confidence will grow. Each training cycle forms the foundation for the next training cycle. So, if you have ambitious goals, understand that your training for a goal could begin years before you reach it. Each step leads you closer as subsequent months build on previous months.

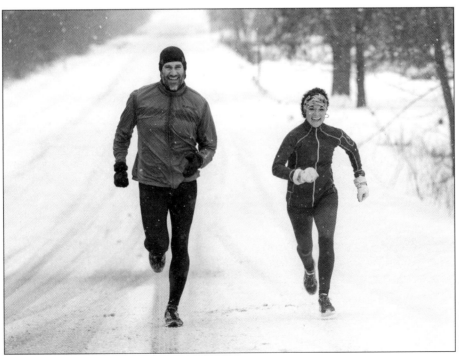

Next, your goals need to be things that you really want. Goals that matter to you and that you will work for. They're goals that will get you out the door when you'd rather sleep in. Goals that will get you doing that strength work today that you want to put off until tomorrow, and the tomorrow after that. They are the goals that will get you pushing and resting harder when needed.

Goals also need to be measurable. Saying "I want to get faster" or "I want to be able to run longer" or "I want to be stronger"—all these goals are too vague. You need to be able to (a) measure progress along the way, and (b) know when you've reached your goal. There is no way to ever reach vague goals that have no end. However, if you say, "I want to run a sub-30-minute 5K in six months," here you have a specific, measurable goal. You can track your progress along the way, which provides encouragement and fuels your desire. You know when you're on target and when you are not. And you've set a deadline, so you're less likely to procrastinate and find excuses for not doing what you know you need to do to achieve your goal.

Age Grading

Age grading allows for a comparison of performances across age and sex. It levels the playing field, in a sense, for older athletes. At 55, 65, or 75, you can plug your time into an age-grade calculator, and it will tell you your equivalent time at age 25 (your so-called ideal time). Age-grade tables were first introduced in 1989 by the World Association of Veteran Athletes (now World Masters Athletics), the world's governing body for masters track and field, and are continually updated to reflect changing results.

What is the advantage of age grading? Well, it's a bit like assigning a handicap in golf, though this doesn't reflect ability but rather normal physiological changes that all runners must deal with at some point. It allows older runners to know where they really stand against younger competitors. For many, you see that in reality you are still setting PRs and can continue to do so for decades to come.

Empirically, age grading does seem to work. Many longtime athletes will notice that their age-graded times are fairly consistent with the actual times they posted when they were younger. You can use this calculation to compare yourself today with your younger self (and vice versa), and you can compare your performance to that of other runners of any age.

While few races in the United States determine race results via age grading (this is done more often outside the United States), it's an interesting tool for runners to play with. Along with age-group awards, age grading makes it possible for competitive runners to keep pursuing ambitious race results.

When choosing goals, it's best to consider both reality and dreams. Having dreams is great, but if those dreams are so grand that you feel forever discouraged, then you are more likely to just give up. In chapter 4, I will offer some specific guidelines on how to determine reasonable goals and how to organize an annual training plan that will help you reach them.

Finding Your Greatness

One problem I see with runners—and this applies to all ages but can really undermine the progress and enjoyment of older runners—is that you can get caught up in the numbers, measuring and remeasuring yourself against others and even comparing your current self to your younger self. As C.S. Lewis aptly put it, "Comparison is the thief of joy." Comparison is hard to avoid and important to address. It's likely that you do it to some degree. You want community; you want to share your stories and adventures with those who share your passions. You want to inspire and be inspired. But when you see others doing amazing things, does that inspire you to also take on big things, whatever that may be for you, or does it make you feel smaller? When you look at what you've done in the past, does that make you feel more capable, or does it make you feel like nothing but a shell of your former self?

Returning to my story about Aristotle in chapter 1, let's suppose you want to live your best life: You want to flourish now and always. Remember, this is a *process* of being. It's not something you achieve once and then you get to coast for the rest of your life. Achievement in the past only matters if it leads to a full and excellent life throughout the years. The classic story of the high school football star who lives forever in the past, reminiscing on the good old days when he was young and strong and happy, is not what you're after here. Likewise, if you feel you've somehow not lived a flourishing life in the past, that does not mean you cannot change the story starting now. You can still achieve your greatness, whatever that is, and it's up to you to define it and create it.

An excellent human being, a person who is living a good life for and as a human, exercises human virtues. Virtues are those admirable characteristics that suffer neither deficiency nor excess. So courage is a mathematical mean of action, where one feels just the right amount of fear—not too much and not too little. But here's the catch with courage: The courageous act in any situation is not the same for everyone. It's also not relative. For me, given who I am, my skills, my genetic gifts and handicaps, the courageous act is one specific action; I just have to figure out what that action is. And it will be a different action from the courageous act for you, because you are a different person with different skills and genetic strengths and weaknesses. But for you, there is also only one right action. And then there is the situation. Every situation is different. Each individual and each situation yield one right action.

Let's suppose you're standing on the beach. The surf is rough and dark, with menacing waves rolling in fast and furious. You see someone flailing about in the water, calling out for help. You don't know how to swim. Should you attempt to save the person? Well, given your ability, it would be foolhardy of you to wade in after the drowning swimmer. Likewise, it would be cowardly to simply run away in fear or become hysterical. In this situation, you have to ask: What is the rational thing to do, given the situation and my abilities?

Now let's suppose you are an experienced swimmer and a certified lifeguard. This situation is significantly different because *you* are different. Everyone has a mean of action—an absolute that is relative to you—but that mean varies from person to person depending on their skills and strengths, their experience, and even their physical makeup. And this will also vary over a lifetime.

What does this have to do with finding your greatness and your flourishing life? Well, your greatness and your happiness are your own. Your greatness is where you push yourself, given your particular situation, not compared to anyone else or even yourself at a different time. Your greatness today is not about 30 years ago—it's about today. Your greatness is not about what others do—it's about what you do. Your greatness is about finding what makes *your* spine tingle when you think about it and then going after it.

Today, runners are busy completely upending what was previously believed to be possible for older athletes. You're learning that you don't have to give up the things you love just because you reach a certain age. You don't have to fear starting something completely new. It's never too late to start, and you can continue for as long as your creative mind allows. And for those who have been running for years, pursuing goals remains attainable and important as you get older. Likewise, continuing to do something you have benefited from for so long doesn't change over time. Your goals may change relative to where you are in life or just shift in interest or priority, but that is irrespective of age.

A 2018 study following male runners from the age of 45 to 95 found that there was a linear decline in race times of about 1 percent per year up to the late 70s (Fair and Kaplan). After that, the decline increased significantly, but this certainly suggests that things do not go downhill as quickly as previously believed. Many still believe that your ability to run either faster or longer declines precipitously after your mid to late 30s, but both anecdotal examples and research indicate that this is not the case. Study after study clearly shows that remaining active significantly slows the normal decline as you age but doesn't render it nonexistent.

In a study of 415,000 masters runners above 50, marathon participation increased at a greater rate than in younger age groups, and the top masters runners improved their marathon times at a faster rate than younger runners. What this means is that the top marathoners show an improvement in average marathon times, and this improvement is seen to a greater extent in older athletes. The number of masters athletes running marathons is also increasing faster than other age groups (Jokl, Sethi, and Cooper 2004). This shows that the limits for older athletes may be well beyond what you've reached thus far.

This matters not just for those who wish to test themselves competitively but also for those who want to continue running or begin running for their physical and mental health and for social reasons as they age. These studies don't just show that performance declines more gradually up to the age of 70 but also that running slows the declines you often see with aging. So, that's good news, whether you want to keep racing competitively or keep running to retain a vibrant and active life.

Chapter 3

Adapt to Change: Addressing the Needs of Female Runners

Not so long ago, menopause was simply not talked about. Even books written for female athletes often either ignored this stage in every woman's life or offered only a cursory mention of it. There's still very little good research on menopause and its effects for female athletes. However, over the past couple decades, participation in running has steadily increased for women over 50. With that, interest in the effects of menopause has increased, and data has also become more available.

But it's important to recognize that our understanding of this stage in a woman's life is just beginning. In many cases, we may not yet know the underlying mechanisms leading to the effects often observed before, during, and after menopause. Most research focuses on the decline in estrogen and then infers that this is the cause of observable changes. The challenge is to understand the how of menopause so you can address those more difficult changes.

This chapter will look at exercise, recovery, and nutrition in light of this life transition. While some research is now being conducted on female-specific issues, it is still in its infancy. Most advice available today is extrapolated from the basic understanding of what happens physiologically and hormonally during different stages of a woman's life and cycle. This can help address some common concerns, but being in tune with how your body responds to exercise, nutrition, and recovery is the most important awareness you can develop as an older athlete. Women in particular must train based on their unique needs in order to pursue goals, take on new adventures, and become happier and healthier.

For women entering their 50s and beyond, the challenges of perimenopause, menopause, and postmenopause are real, but it does not mean the end of a woman's athletic life. In fact, menopause can present new opportunities, and in many cases, running can help women transition through menopause more smoothly.

Understanding Hormonal Changes

While there is no one answer to when perimenopause begins, it is usually identified via a woman's subjective experience of certain symptoms such as irregular periods, hot flashes, and night sweats. This is a time when the ovaries gradually stop producing eggs, resulting in hormone fluctuations and unpredictable cycles. Perimenopause often begins in the late 30s or early 40s and continues into the late 40s to mid-50s. Menopause is marked as the point when 12 months have passed following a woman's last menstrual period.

It's important, from the outset, to understand that perimenopause and menopause are experienced differently by every woman. Just like any other phase of a woman's life, how and when each woman experiences it varies based on genetics, environment, prior training, and other factors. Recent research focusing on how hormones fluctuate during a woman's reproductive years helps us understand how to adjust for and address the effects of these cyclical changes; but with perimenopause and menopause, this cyclical predictability disappears. Anecdotally, 80 to 90 percent of women cite related physical and mental difficulties, including hot flashes or night sweats, sexual dysfunction, depression, brain fog, irritability, and sleep disturbances (Grant et al. 2015). Menopause also brings a reduction in muscle strength and mass, an increased risk for cardiovascular disease and stroke, a decline in protein synthesis (which you need to build muscle), and a gradual decrease in bone density.

While getting through the transition can present serious challenges, many female runners welcome the end of their monthly cycles. If this next stage of life is welcomed and embraced, rather than dreaded and feared, both seeing the advantages and addressing the challenges, this time can reveal new paths of opportunity. Based on life expectancy, women spend more than a third of their lives postmenopausal. If this stage is going to be lived well—healthy, active, and mentally vibrant—it's necessary to know how to address potential changes. It is estimated that between 80 and 90 percent of women experience physical and psychological menopausal symptoms ranging from mild to severe. Physical activity, such as running, may reduce these symptoms while also addressing more general age-related decline (Dąbrowska et al. 2016).

As research continues to explore the changes that happen during menopause, many women now feel empowered to know that what they are experiencing is not just in their head—something women are often told. At the same rate, women should not be discouraged or feel doomed; the undesirable symptoms they may be dealing with now will not continue for the rest of their lives. Women in perimenopause and menopause can address many of the symptoms they experience, some of which may change over time. Additionally, not every changing symptom a woman faces at this time of life is necessarily related to menopause. Finally, it is very important to understand and accept that all women are individuals and will experience these changes differently. Some will have more symptoms than others. Some may not even notice any changes. It's important to pay attention to your lived experience and seek out solutions to the specific challenges you face.

While hormones keep you healthy and allow you to adapt to stress, including exercise, hormonal changes also present challenges as you age. Specifically, human growth hormone, testosterone, and estrogen decline with age. Human growth hormone (HGH) is crucial for the recovery and repair of tissues, and testosterone and estrogen are anabolic hormones that help you adapt and grow stronger in response to exercise stress. The effects of these hormonal changes include the following:

Decreased Training Response

Cardiovascular and energy systems respond less efficiently because of lower estrogen, which is the primary anabolic hormone for women. During this time, using the estrogen that is available becomes more important. For this reason, adding some high intensity work is beneficial for menopausal and postmenopausal women. Maintaining aerobic work is significant for cardiovascular health. While women have a lower risk of cardiovascular disease prior to menopause, this risk increases significantly after menopause, suggesting that estrogen provides a protective advantage for women.

Changes in Body Composition

Over time, it becomes more difficult to maintain muscle mass, and fat distribution shifts. This applies to aging in general, but as estrogen drops, women must change the way they train to make the most of what they've got. Estrogen plays a role in metabolism, and as it declines, fat tends to store itself around the belly, which is more typical for men. The balance of protein synthesis (which builds muscle) and protein breakdown (which uses muscle for energy) also shifts, with breakdown outpacing synthesis. More fat and less muscle makes it more difficult to maintain strength, speed, and power. The good news is that with some tweaking of your training, adding in more intensity and strength, you can counteract a lot of the changes that may present challenges (Figueroa et al. 2003).

Loss of Musculoskeletal Tissue Quality

Muscles, tendons, ligaments, and bones are all more prone to injury during menopause because menopause brings a drastic reduction in estrogen, making this a more serious problem for women. But proper training and recovery can offset this. Exercise, adequate protein and carbohydrate intake, and possibly some supplements can help attenuate the loss of muscle and bone mass and improve joint mobility and the quality of connective tissue.

Decreased Sleep Quality

As I've discussed before, sleep is when you repair, rebuild, and get stronger. Sleep is when HGH is most active. Unfortunately, sleep disturbances are one of the major complaints for women throughout the perimenopause-postmenopause continuum. Here, the decline in both progesterone and estrogen has an impact on sleep quality, respiration, body temperature, deep sleep, and the ability to fall asleep quickly and stay asleep.

Increased Mental Health Issues

Activity supports mental health as much as physical health. Our brains are physical, so the physical changes that occur during menopause affect the brain as much as the rest of the body. During perimenopause and beyond, many women report mental health issues, including anxiety, forgetfulness, brain fog, anger, depression, mood swings, low self-esteem, and irritability. Many studies show a relationship between physical activity and improved mental health and quality of life. It's not surprising that this also applies to menopause (Elavsky and McAuley 2007). While the decline in estrogen leads to a reduction in serotonin (a mood-regulating neurotransmitter), exercise increases serotonin. Serotonin also works with melatonin to regulate sleep. The combination results in improved mood regulation and well-being.

Declining Bone Density

Women reach their peak bone density in their early 30s. After that, it gradually declines until late perimenopause or during menopause, when the decline become precipitous for about five to seven years. Genetics, environment, activity, and nutrition all play a role in maintaining bone density, but the decline in estrogen greatly impacts bone density as well. It's important to understand how bone health is maintained in order to counteract this process.

As with muscle, bones build and break down. Bone remodeling involves osteoclasts and osteoblasts. Osteoclasts break down old bone (bone resorption), a necessary process to maintain bone quality. Osteoblasts build new bone (bone formation). The balance of activity between osteoclasts and osteoblasts is crucial for healthy bone. With the reduction of estrogen, which inhibits bone resorption, bone breaks down faster than it builds back up. The aim is to mitigate the rate at which bone breaks down.

Ideally, you want to have excellent bone density at the time of peak density in your early 30s because that will give you the best chance of avoiding serious osteoporosis, but there are still things you can do during menopause to reduce bone loss. Exercise that stresses bone through mechanical loading—running, lifting, jumping—encourages the activity of osteoblasts (Ji et al. 2023). The body only maintains what it needs based on the demands made of it. If you aren't making physical demands, then your body will not use precious resources to maintain those structures. The saying "use it or lose it" applies to bone just as much as to muscle, but without a strong skeleton, you cannot have strong muscles.

Counteracting Hormonal Changes

All this could leave you feeling pretty pessimistic and discouraged. In many cases, a third of a woman's life is lived postmenopause, so it's important to understand what's happening and address it if you want to maintain, or even improve, your quality of life.

Exercise

The overwhelming evidence shows that exercise improves your overall health. Inactivity leads to early decline, and the benefits for women concerning bone density, cardiovascular health, obesity (and its comorbidities), and mental health are particularly compelling. There is also a good bit of research indicating that exercise can help manage some of the symptoms of menopause: anxiety, brain fog, mood issues, poor sleep quality, and low self-esteem (Dąbrowska-Galas et al. 2019). This question remains and continues to be explored: What sort of exercise is best for women moving through the different stages of menopause?

The accepted recommendation for exercise is 150 minutes of moderate exercise weekly. However, studies have suggested that for menopausal and postmenopausal women, a higher dose of exercise may be beneficial (Dalleck et al. 2009). There appears to be a possible dose-response relationship, where an increase in exercise duration improves cardiorespiratory health, body mass and composition, waist circumference, and blood-lipid composition. The evidence clearly points to the benefits of getting regular exercise. But what type, or types, of exercise is most efficacious to attenuate the undesirable effects of menopause?

Strength and Resistance Training

It makes a lot of sense for women in this stage of life to be strength training. Why? First, strength training counteracts some of the natural decline in bone density and muscle mass and strength that comes with aging, some of which men also experience. Second, women may start losing the anabolic effects of estrogen—and some testosterone, though that plays a smaller role throughout a woman's life in most cases—but they still have some, and they need to use it as efficiently as possible.

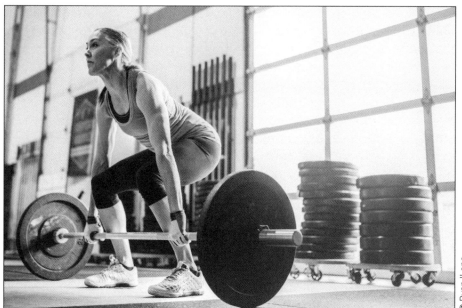

The problem is that as you get older, you tend to stop focusing on the things you actually need to keep in your tool belt. Traditionally, women have shied away from strength. Gender stereotypes and concerns about developing bulky muscles lead women to either avoid lifting or, if they do lift, focus on high repetitions and lower weights. Of course, this is not always the case, but if this applies to you, I am challenging you to shake things up. More evidence is emerging that women need to lift heavier weights because that makes the most of the limited estrogen available. Here, heavier weights mean those you can lift for no more than 8 to 12 repetitions and repeat for about three sets.

It is worth noting that some recent compelling studies found that powerlifting produces better results than strength training (Stengel et al. 2005). The difference between powerlifting and strength training is the velocity of the concentric part of the lift. For example, let's look at a basic bicep curl. A powerlifting version of a bicep curl would spend one second in the concentric phase (curl) and four seconds in the eccentric phase (lower). A strength-training version of a bicep curl would involve a four-second curl and a four-second lower. However, powerlifting increases stress—and with that, the likelihood of injury—so it is best done in low doses. The combination of a low dose of powerlifting along with moderate doses of strength training appears to offer the best results for bone health and muscle strength. Low to moderate load, high-velocity resistance training has been seen to improve muscle composition and strength, power output, functional abilities, and bone health. It is believed that the rate of loading and unloading is likely responsible for the greater osteogenic response and that there is greater demand on different types of muscle fibers and neuromuscular activation. For those dealing with early osteoporosis or osteopenia, this presents some very promising options.

But any strength work helps, and like anything else, you need to start from where you are now. You don't need to go to a gym to do strength work unless you prefer to do so. A couple hand weights, or even a jug of water, will have you ready to start. A stairway or bench makes for great strength work as well. Using your body weight to work against gravity while stepping or running up stairs or a hill increases the demand on your muscles. Just walk up a few flights of stairs at a pressing effort, and you will feel your muscles working harder. Stepping up and down a bench in a controlled way also uses your body weight as a strength-building tool. Working up to box jumps as you get stronger turns this into a muscle-building, bone-building, and neurological training exercise. Get creative!

Keep in mind to start slow and progress gradually. Focus on stability and balance exercises first. Then move on to strength and endurance, completing multiple sets of exercises that fatigue targeted muscle groups. Next comes muscular development, which increases the load but reduces repetitions. At this point, you're performing five to seven repetitions and five sets of each exercise. You'll find more guidance about strength work in chapter 6. And finally, heavy lifting and plyometrics can be very beneficial, but they must be done correctly and only once you have progressed to that point. Explosive exercises like jumping (e.g., box jumps) offer huge benefits for joint mobility, fast-twitch muscle activation, and coordination.

If you are new to lifting or aren't sure when it's appropriate to add more challenging exercises, a few sessions with a personal trainer may be helpful. A personal trainer can assess where you're at now, identify overactive or underactive muscles, observe movement patterns, and then provide you with a plan that will address your strengths and weaknesses.

Aerobic Training

While easy aerobic exercise is still important, adding some intensity to your running is necessary to keep your body strong and able to handle the demands of your training. Like with lifting, women have traditionally not been encouraged to add intensity to their exercise. Since many women 50 and over have come to running without a lot of experience in sports, they are often encouraged to stick with walking, yoga, Pilates, and light lifting—such as high repetitions with low weights. In running, these women are often recommended to do light jogging over hard sprinting and hill work. Not so long ago, women were told that running would cause their uteruses to fall out. That legacy has left many women over 50 wondering how to even begin.

An example of adding intensity is to do steep hill repeats, which offer fantastic strength work and improve your speed and mobility. These need not be overly taxing. Find a short, steep hill. Try to run hard, or even walk fast, for 8 to 10 seconds, then recover for 10 seconds, and repeat this 5 to 10 times. These intensity bursts should not be longer than 10 seconds because longer bouts may compromise quality.

Another way to add intensity is to throw in some short strides at the end of your easy runs to encourage neuromuscular development. In fact, these can be added at the end of every run—just add five or so fast surges for 10 to 20 seconds each. Go to the track and run 100-meter sprint-floats. This is one of my favorite workouts because it's fun. The idea is to sprint on the straightaways and "float" the turns. After an easy 10- to 15-minute warm-up, try 5 to 10 of these sprint-floats. Over time, do as many as you can until your form starts to break down.

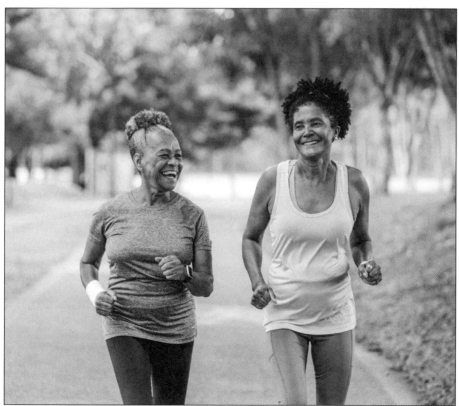

© Andreswd

> ## Hormone Replacement Therapy
>
> For some women, hormone replacement therapy (HRT) is something to consider and discuss with their doctor. All women are individuals, and each one experiences menopause differently. When quality of life becomes an issue due to poor sleep, brain fog, depression, anxiety, or other symptoms, HRT may be your best option. Additionally, if you continue running and exercising, you can mitigate some of the risks of HRT—like the slight increase in the chances of getting breast cancer.
>
> What's important to keep in mind is that menopause is not a time of deficiency. It's not a state of disease or decay or decline. Menopause is not a condition. HRT can help women move through the transition if they have issues that are difficult to manage, but it's not replacing some deficiency. Menopause is natural. Aging is natural. How are you going to age?

Nutrition

This is a time when good nutrition really counts. Since women do not synthesize protein as well postmenopause, quality protein is crucial. Taking in protein before and after exercise and before bed can help with muscle mass, sleep, and, as a result, recovery. Calcium, magnesium, vitamin D, vitamin K_2, and collagen are all essential for bone health—along with exercise that stresses the bones. Melatonin helps regulate the sleep cycle, which results in better recovery and rejuvenation.

Recovery

As I said in chapter 1, sleep is your most important recovery tool. Sleep allows for adaptation to happen faster. HGH is released when you sleep. Eating a little protein before sleep also encourages further recovery and adaptation and has been shown to improve sleep quality. The discussion of sleep and sleep quality has weaved itself throughout this entire chapter because it really is that important. Good sleep plus good nutrition is central to recovery and, thus, becoming stronger after menopause. Addressing sleep issues and increasing protein intake in addition to other recommended recovery protocols (discussed in chapter 7) will have you recovering well, pursuing your goals and desires, and feeling excited and motivated.

While menopause can present challenges for female athletes, it's important to understand that on all counts, continuing to run can make things better. While you do need to change a few things, you can keep pursuing your athletic goals. Menopause is just another phase.

The medical and scientific establishment has been dominated by men and socially constructed assumptions concerning women's bodies. Let's not forget that it was not so long ago that the medical establishment believed a woman's uterus would fall out if she ran more than a 10K. Menopause, like menstruation, has been and continues to be shrouded in social constructions and gender stereotypes. Assumptions concerning aging in general can have a negative effect as well, which makes aging as a woman that much more difficult.

Those of you who want something more are on the cutting edge of big changes. I've witnessed this change over the past 20 years or so. Women in their 50s, 60s, 70s, and beyond are breaking records, setting new high points, and doing things no one believed possible. And this is just the beginning. Of course, this applies to older athletes in general who are reaching athletic goals that seemed impossible just a decade ago. But for women in particular, who only 50 years ago had very limited athletic opportunities, the gains are spectacular. The women who follow will stand on the shoulders of the female athletes of today. You are an inspiration. Of course, living life on your own terms—demanding solutions and answers to the challenges you face during this stage in life—means you can continue to enjoy the things you always have and even explore new adventures and goals.

PART II

TRAINING

Chapter 4

Identifying the Building Blocks of Successful Training

Many runners, both novice and experienced, end up doing a lot of cutting and pasting when it comes to training. I refer to this as "noodling around." You take a workout from one recommended plan that you like parts of and another workout from another plan you like and plug them into your calendar. You read magazine articles and social media posts about a cool new workout, so you add it too. The logic seems to go like this: If I just take the best training runs from each approach, I'll have a killer program. Of course, it might just kill your running too, or at least injure you. Some runners stick with the plan they've used for years, even if it's not working, maybe switching up some things here and there—but without understanding what they should be adding and changing. Runners ask me questions like "Should I just add some miles to the plan I'm already using?" That's also what I call noodling—you tweak the plan without taking all the variables into account. You can't just take a given plan and add miles to it and call it a better plan. You also can't just take a plan and add more speed to get faster.

You should follow certain principles in training, taking into account what you are training for and your end goal, both of which are aimed at maximizing your body's response and making it stronger, faster, and better at running—no matter your age.

Using Periodization to Plan Your Training

A key part of smart training is periodization: dividing your year into distinct periods to focus on different training variables and work toward short-term goals with long-term goals in mind. This means you'll do different things at different points in your training. Periodization maximizes desired training adaptations over time while preventing stagnation or overtraining. Periodization allows you to use your goals as a guide to develop different aspects of fitness at different times, and this is helpful whether you race or not and whether you run 5Ks, marathons, or ultramarathons. Since different types of training stimulus bring different adaptations, periodization allows you to fully develop your neuromuscular and metabolic systems by tapping into different stimuli at different times during training, along with progressive overload (gradual increase in stress). Macrocycles, mesocycles, and microcycles are key organizational elements of any good periodized plan (see figure 4.1). Let's take a closer look:

> **Periodization** allows you to use your goals as a guide to develop different aspects of fitness at different times, and this is helpful whether you race or not and whether you run 5Ks, marathons, or ultramarathons.

- *Macrocycle:* A macrocycle is basically a set time frame that includes shorter cycles or phases (described below). It is the longest cycle of training and could be a year (or more), six months, three months, or less, depending on your goals. The macrocycle is often broken up into several phases:
  - *Preparation:* This is foundational training completed prior to goal-specific training, and it's the first step in planning and preparing for goals. Preparation is done prior to starting a focused training block or during the early weeks of a training block.
  - *Competition:* This is goal-specific training. As you get closer to your goal, such as a race, specific training becomes more important to allow for the adaptations you will need to achieve your goal.
  - *Transition or offseason:* This is your annual or semiannual recovery phase between focused training blocks or your annual deloading period. How long these last will depend on the distances you are training for. For instance, the time between marathon training cycles will often be longer than the time between 5K training cycles.
- *Mesocycle:* Within each macrocycle are mesocycles, which often focus on different elements such as aerobic development, strength or hill training, speed progression, or race-specific training. How long these last will vary, but they usually fall within four to eight weeks. Four weeks is typical, but depending on the goal and how you're responding to the training, this can change.
- *Microcycle:* The shortest phase of training is the microcycle, which falls within a mesocycle and covers daily and weekly training goals. Microcycles are usually between 7 and 10 days long.

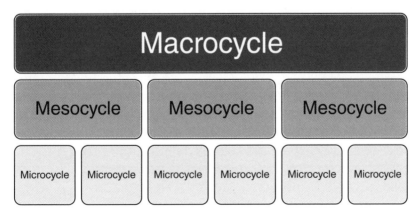

FIGURE 4.1 Key elements of periodization.

As an example, let's say the macrocycle is a marathon training program of 18 weeks. That macrocycle can then be broken up into several mesocycles, such as base building, hill work, and speed. Then each microcycle will present the weekly detail, setting out daily workouts with the specific mesocycle focus in mind. This allows you to create an organized plan, a road map of sorts, that focuses on the different adaptations needed for the goal you're training for.

When training, you must understand that you cannot do everything all at the same time. Doing so can cause injuries and suboptimal training because you're focusing on everything and, as a result, are not able to do anything very well. I see this happen time and again in running groups, where everyone runs hills on Tuesdays, track intervals on Thursdays, and long runs on Saturdays—and they do this year-round, week after week. This approach is unlikely to help you progress your fitness and running abilities, whereas periodized training allows you to both focus your workouts based on your goals and allows for adequate recovery.

Just as different phases (macrocycle, mesocycle, and microcycle) of training have different purposes, there are also different ways to organize these phases. Two common types of plans are linear and block periodization, and you can use one or the other depending on your needs.

The classical, or linear, approach develops multiple areas simultaneously with a modest increase in those variables. The general rule is to increase your net stress no more than 10 percent weekly, but this rule does not always apply. While the 10-percent rule may be a safe increase, those who are doing less to begin with can often add a bit more. So, if you are currently running 8 miles a week, the 10-percent rule means that next week you can increase to 8.8 miles. At this level, you can likely go up to 10 miles. But consider the runner who is running 60 miles. Adding 10 percent means increasing to 66 miles. That seems reasonable, while 70 miles might be too much. So the 10-percent rule tends to work better once you are running more than 30 miles a week.

Importantly, you do not want to add different elements of training at the same time. If you add aerobic volume, do not also add more speed. If you add more speed, hold aerobic volume steady. Only increase one element at a time. You might start with an endurance mesocycle of three to five weeks—or more, because you can always build more aerobic endurance—then add hills while slightly reducing endurance for the next mesocycle, then add speed while slightly reducing endurance and hills. The overall volume of stress increases modestly since the increase is only in one area, which means that this is a fairly safe approach to training, especially for a novice runner. The drawback is a lack of specific focus, so the gains in any particular area are limited.

A block approach focuses on developing one training stimulus at a time. You might have an endurance phase, a hill phase, and a speed phase, for example. While other aspects of training are still part of the plan, the focus in a block plan is on overloading a specific stimulus. Typically, this type of training is organized into four-week mesocycles, where the fourth week is a recovery week that allows your body to rebuild and respond to the increasing demands. For block periodization, the mesocycle either starts high and progresses lower (in volume or intensity) or starts low and progresses higher. The aim in both cases is accumulated fatigue. For example, in a block endurance mesocycle, a plan will either add volume over the three-week build and then drop back for the fourth week or begin the cycle with a higher volume and then reduce that slightly for the following two weeks and end with the fourth week as a recovery, or unloading, week. Remember that with a block plan, you will not add other stresses; speed, hills, and other areas will be held constant or reduced.

Different plans work for different runners. Classical, or linear, periodization tends to work better for less experienced runners because the loads are more modest, reducing some of the risk of overdoing it, but the gains are also more modest. Block periodization can result in greater fitness gains, but the risks of overreach, injury, and excessive fatigue require careful monitoring and adjustment—and this can pose additional risks for older runners, who may need more recovery time and more modest increases. For runners 50 and over, training plans that emphasize fitness over fatigue are preferable because too much fatigue can require additional recovery time. Training will cause some temporary fatigue, but pushing too far leads to injury and lost training time. Any lost training time undermines consistency.

The plans found in part III are modified and responsive—they can be adjusted based on how you are responding—block periodization plans, where one stimulus is added at a time and increases are modest over a mesocycle, with ample recovery included in the microcycles (weeks). They progressively increase in specificity based on the race being trained for. If you're training for a 5K, that means building your aerobic base first and then increasing race-specific speed. If you're training for a marathon, and assuming you have the necessary aerobic base, that means working on speed development early on and then increasing marathon-paced runs and long runs later in the training.

It's important to keep these things in mind when you choose a training plan:

- It should work for your life. Find something you can do given other life demands.

- It should introduce a new stimulus gradually. If you see sudden jumps in intensity or volume, avoid those plans.
- It should include recovery periods. If you see continuous weeks of high or increasing volume or intensity without rest periods, avoid those plans.
- It should move from less race-specific to more race-specific.
- It should allow for adjustments based on how you're responding. This is difficult with a pre-prepared plan, and it's one reason I rarely recommend them. But personal coaching is not an option for everyone, so understanding how and when to adjust is important as a self-coached runner.

Aligning Training With Your Goals

Once you've established a robust aerobic base of fitness, how should your training build on that? The how depends on your specific short-, medium-, and long-term goals. As I've said repeatedly, running offers infinite options concerning goals. However, there are reasonable and unreasonable progressions and goal combinations. Goals ideally build on one another, just as microcycles build on each other within a mesocycle, and mesocycles build on each other within a macrocycle. Part of planning your periodization is setting goals. These goals can be organized into an annual plan or an even longer period. You might have a goal of running a marathon in two years. What should you do to get yourself there? If you're new to running, your plan will look different than if you've been running for several years or decades. Let's look at a few examples:

> **Running** offers infinite options concerning goals. However, there are reasonable and unreasonable progressions and goal combinations.

- *Example 1:* Over the course of a year, you may have goals within a macrocycle, building from a 5K mesocycle to a 10K mesocycle to a half-marathon mesocycle. That annual plan or macrocycle can then be the base for a progression to a marathon the following year or for setting more ambitious time goals for the distances you have been training for.
- *Example 2:* You have a burning desire to see how fast you can run a 5K. You've been working on your aerobic base, and now you want to add in some speed work. You've signed up for several 5Ks over the next few months. You want to plan your training so that you peak before each race, ideally peaking a bit higher each time.

- *Example 3:* You've just gotten into trail running and are thinking about running an ultra. You've run several road marathons over the years, and now you want to see how far you can really go. You pick a local trail 50K with some fairly technical running and decent climbing. You wonder how best to take your road-running fitness and transition to new demands.

When thinking about goals, you want to consider what your primary goal is. You can set multiple goals along the way, and those can be used as fitness benchmarks or stand-alone goals. As an example: Many runners target a goal of running a marathon in the spring and the fall. But what do they do when they aren't specifically training for one of those marathons? You can set mini goals between training cycles. These mini goals can serve two very important functions: (1) they keep you motivated, and (2) they focus on areas that need improvement. And they can be just as exciting and fulfilling as those bigger goals that so many runners fixate on.

If you're a novice runner looking to run your first 5K, 10K, half-marathon, or beyond, you can set smaller goals that work you up to this long-term goal. This is not just about fitness; it's also about learning how to deal with race situations, logistics, and problems that inevitably pop up during races—and just getting comfortable being in a situation where you have goals and might feel pressure.

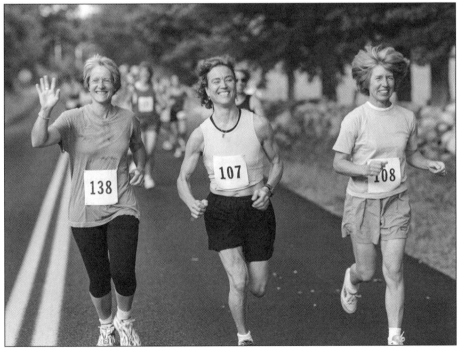

Also note that when setting goals, it's important to look at your experience, where you are now, and where you want to be in the future. Of course, your plans can change, but starting where you are and aiming for something reasonable now will lead you to the next step, whatever that may be. As you travel down new roads, previously unknown paths may reveal themselves. Let's say you start off with a couch-to-5K program. At the time, your one goal is to run a 5K. You start running regularly, feel yourself getting stronger, run the 5K, and actually enjoy it. You find yourself thinking about a 10K, which just three months ago would have seemed unfathomable, but now it seems possible. Perhaps

What's Your Athletic Age?

Athletic age is a concept used in coaching to determine where an athlete is in their athletic development. This is different from biological age, and it's something coaches use whether you're a 16-year-old high school runner or a 60-year-old aspiring marathoner. Athletic age concerns how many years you've been active in any sport. Obviously, some sports will overlap with running more than others; if you've been cycling for years, that will figure in more than if you've been rock climbing for years—but both count.

If you haven't been active in a sport consistently, then you are very young in terms of athletic age. This has both benefits and drawbacks. The main benefit is the potential for improvement. In running, most see steady improvement in both fitness and outcomes (race times, distances, etc.) for about 10 years, then those improvements tend to level off. You can still improve, but those improvements are generally in smaller increments. So, for those who are newer to the sport, maybe even discovering running at 50 or over, you have the potential to see improvement for quite some time. The drawback is that you need to first develop your foundation, which may mean a longer developmental period and more short-term goals leading up to long-term goals.

For those who have been running for a while, say 10 years or more, there are also pluses and minuses: A plus is that you have a deep fitness foundation to draw on to tackle big goals soon. A minus is that improvement requires very smart and purposeful training that targets your particular strengths and weaknesses. Since you likely have a good aerobic base, you may now need to add more specific speed work (tempos, intervals, or repeats) and hill work or learn how to pace well. You tend to do what you're good at because you tend to *like* doing what you're good at. But at this point, you will gain more by working on the things you're not so good at. Do not shy away from the things that challenge you the most, even when it can be humbling and maybe even discouraging. With any training plan, you will have runs that push you in ways that may feel uncomfortable, but that's where you find progress, and the uncomfortable will become more comfortable.

you think, "Maybe I can run a 5K faster." Or you even think, "Maybe I can do a half-marathon next year." All these new paths have been revealed because you traveled down the couch-to-5K road.

Annual plans need not be etched in stone. They can be edited along the way based on how things are going and if your desires change, but they must be dictated by where you are right now. If you run your first 5K and then think about running a marathon in two months, the result is likely to disappoint.

Goals in running can be whatever you want. If you run, you are a runner, whether it's 100 meters or 100 miles.

One thing to keep in mind about goals is that farther does not necessarily mean better. You may believe you aren't a real runner unless you've run a marathon. Goals in running can be whatever you want. If you run, you are a runner, whether it's 100 meters or 100 miles. The crucial part when thinking about an annual plan is that you aim for goals you deeply care about and that are based on where you are in your running journey right now.

The Five Principles of Solid Training

Wherever you are in your running journey, the principles of training apply to everyone. Be mindful of these five training principles:

1. Foundation of aerobic conditioning
2. Responsive training
3. Perceived effort
4. Progressive and sequential development
5. Tapering and peaking

Foundation of Aerobic Conditioning

Chapter 5 will go into this in greater depth, but all aerobic running (any run longer than 400 meters) begins with building your aerobic engine. This is just like the foundation of a house. If you build your house on a foundation of cinder blocks, it won't be as strong as a house built on a deep and strong foundation. The deeper the foundation, the taller you can build your house, adding all the floors for injury resistance, longevity, endurance, training tolerance, speed, and strength.

Responsive Training

I call this "training responsively," which means you adjust your training based on how you're responding, concerning both improvements and recovery. Let's say that this week you aim to run a long run of 10 miles at a pace of 10:00 minutes per mile. During the run, your effort level feels very hard, and you spend the rest of the day on the couch feeling completely wiped out. Or say you set out to do a speed workout that calls for 6 x 800 meters at a pace you just can't seem to hit. How should you respond to this feedback? Let's add that your heart rate remains elevated for a long time after the run, and you still feel sore and have low energy two days later.

In this case, responsive training calls for a close analysis. Are you usually able to complete these runs? If so, this may just be an exception. Individual bad runs are not necessarily cause for concern, but if you see a trend happening—you're constantly sore and tired and unable to complete your workouts—then that calls for an adjustment based on how you're responding to the training. Perhaps you're setting paces that are currently too fast for you. Or maybe you are going into these runs too tired, which is a recovery or training issue.

Perceived Effort

Learning to feel and tap into your Rate of Perceived Effort (RPE), how you feel when you are running, is one of the most important skills a runner needs to develop. You shouldn't just rely on data from technology but also learn to tap into how you're feeling—both when you're running and when you're not running—how you're recovering, and whether you're working hard all the time or not hard enough.

The trick with recovery days is that you should feel better and be recovered for your next hard run, not necessarily your easy run.

One of the common complaints I hear from runners is that their easy recovery days feel the worst. You would think an easy run would feel—well, easy—but that's not necessarily how it works. The trick with recovery days is that you should feel better and be recovered for your next hard run, not necessarily your easy run. The easy run may feel sluggish. You may feel a bit heavy or achy starting out. Ideally, a recovery run should end with you feeling a little better, but it's really the next day that the easy run matters because that next day is when you'll feel ready to take on a harder or longer run.

Progressive and Sequential Development

This principle means that you train with a purpose. You can go out and run and maybe just see how you feel and wing it a bit, but that doesn't develop you physically or mentally for anything specific.

I ran for years and years just doing what I felt like doing that day, and that worked fine for me. But when I returned to racing, that didn't work any longer. I had goals that I needed to train my body more specifically for. Goals don't need to be races, but if you have any goals, it helps to find the most direct path to reach them. Sure, you can take a circuitous route, but it's going to take a lot longer, or you might miss the goal entirely.

Crossing the Grand Canyon and running a fast 5K are very different goals, and each will dictate how your training should proceed. You might still want to do some fast running when training for the Grand Canyon, but that would be something you do early in your training. Later, you will focus on increasing weekly running volume and adding in a good bit of climbing. For that fast 5K, however, the longer stuff should come earlier, and the short, fast stuff should be the focus closer to the race.

In terms of progressive, sequential training, you want to focus on two important principles:

1. Concentrate on your weaknesses and the skills that are the least specific to the goal early in the training.
2. As the race or goal gets closer, your training should be more specific to the race or goal.

How you organize your training to allow yourself to peak is also important. Training should ideally bring you to an optimal fitness level for where you are at that time; you are reaching a peak for that cycle. For something like a marathon, your training should all come together on race day. This is one reason it's a really bad idea to run a race-pace long run the week before your race just to test your fitness. The result

Planning Rest and Recovery Periods

Planned rest is necessary for healthy long-term running. Rest should be planned within macrocycles, mesocycles, and microcycles. Examples of rest and recovery periods include the following:

- Recovery weeks can be scheduled into mesocycles. Some runners like to plan a recovery week every fourth week of training.
- Weekly recovery days can be scheduled within microcycles. These can be recovery runs, complete rest, active rest, or cross-training.
- Annual recovery can be scheduled into your annual plan, or macrocycle. An extended recovery time can allow for both a physical and mental recharge period. It does not require complete rest but should include scaled-back volume and possibly some cross-training.

is usually peaking too soon and leaving your best performance on the training course. However, for 5K and even 10K training, you may be able to experience several peaks that build on each other, steadily increasing over the racing season, with the final race as the highest peak. This is certainly a goal in cross-country and track training. If you balance racing with recovery and continued training, you may see steady improvement over a racing season. With shorter races, recovery happens faster, and you can enjoy the fruits of your previous efforts as you continue racing. Of course, that assumes you balance all the elements well.

Tapering and Peaking

Tapering allows your body to absorb and adapt to all the training you've been doing for weeks and months. Many runners look forward to tapering until they are actually tapering—then they feel anxious and antsy. It's not unusual to feel like you've forgotten how to run. Rest assured, you have not forgotten how to run. But it's not easy to balance the need to allow the adaptations to set in and the need to keep fresh.

> **Tapering** allows your body to absorb and adapt to all the training you've been doing for weeks and months.

How long you taper depends on the race and your goals for the race. For a shorter race, a week or so is plenty. Generally, for a marathon or longer, you're looking at a three-week taper. As with everything we've discussed thus far, there are different approaches to tapering. Some runners taper fast from the beginning and then level out. Others taper slowly, progressing to a sharper taper as the race approaches.

One thing there is general agreement on—which doesn't happen often!—is how to balance volume and intensity. During the taper, volume is reduced but intensity is maintained. That means that while your weekly mileage will decrease, you'll still be running pretaper paces. Your aerobic runs will be shorter, and any speed work will be cut in volume, but your paces will stay the same. This approach allows you to get to race day fully adapted to the training but not feeling sluggish.

Peaking is the idea that your training has taken you to the desired fitness level at the right time for your goal or race. This concept is important because sometimes athletes like to test their fitness close to a race, and understanding peaking can help you avoid this mistake. There are many stories of runners, some very experienced and accomplished, who have made this mistake, leading to somewhat disappointing race results. So, if you're feeling fit and have the urge to take it up a notch for your last long run, fight that urge if you want to be ready for the real race.

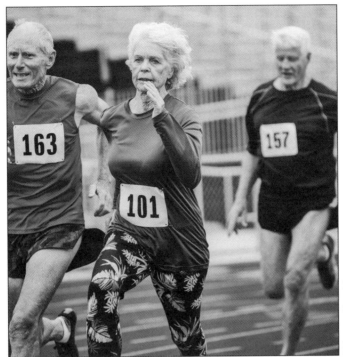

The idea of peaking is also important for training races that you may run along the path to your goal race. If you have a particularly competitive nature and know you won't be able to reel yourself in during a training race (which is usually submaximal), then that training tool is likely a bad one for you. If you can keep your eye on the end goal and use training races well, then they can help you move toward your peak fitness while testing out your race plan and getting more comfortable in a racing environment. Pushing things too hard, too soon, can mean you are past your peak for your goal race. As the saying goes, "Don't leave your race on the training course."

Everything you've learned in this chapter will help guide you in applying the principles of training in a timely and focused manner. Knowing how to organize training for a purpose with your goal as the final aim, while also understanding and embracing the process serves to keep you on track and confident that what you're doing will get you to where you want to be.

You will see all these principles at play in the training plans provided later, but it helps to understand the whys and hows so you can adjust some things based on your goals and your responses. These tools allow you to make smart choices and turn what might otherwise be static training programs into more flexible, individual, and responsive plans. Understanding how to balance stress and recovery, increasing stress slowly and only one variable at a time, allowing for recovery weeks so your body has time to recover and adapt to the training, trading easy days and hard days, responding to how you feel—all these are basic principles to keep in mind to avoid injury, overtraining, burnout, and plateauing. Keep these principles close, and you will reap the benefits of consistent, healthy running.

Chapter 5

Establishing and Maintaining an Aerobic Base

Running any distance longer than 400 meters is primarily an aerobic activity: it requires oxygen to produce energy and relies on the aerobic energy system to generate adenosine triphosphate (ATP), the body's primary source of energy. Aerobic activities typically involve low- to moderate-intensity efforts that can be sustained for extended periods of time. Oxygen is used to break down carbohydrates, fats, and sometimes proteins to produce ATP through a series of metabolic pathways and create the energy we need to continue moving forward. The first step in building running fitness must be establishing what is often referred to as your aerobic engine or aerobic foundation. A robust aerobic system is essential for distance running because it enhances endurance, improves energy utilization, promotes recovery, reduces injury risk, and ultimately leads to greater fitness.

The Importance of an Aerobic Base

This is what I often hear from so many runners, especially older runners who fear that running too much will lead to injury: "I like to run three days a week and cross-train or do CrossFit or high-intensity interval training (HIIT). Less is more, and variety makes you stronger and less prone to injury." If your goal is overall fitness, this approach is fine. If, however, your goal is running—maybe running a marathon or even your first 5K—then specificity rules over everything else. Since this is a book about running, I'm going to concentrate on those of you who are focused on running goals. You cannot escape the empirical reality that if you want to run well, you need to run—and you need to run as much as you can. The exact quantity is very individual, but running needs to be your primary activity if running is your focus.

Here's the classic beginner's marathon program, an approach practiced by novice runners the world over: Run 10 or so total miles during the week (two or three runs for three to four miles each) and then a long run on the weekend—working up to 20 miles, and you may run a couple of those over a 16-week training program. This is a pretty standard approach for many marathon training programs. If your aim is to finish, then this might work—but chances are very good that you will end up injured, never making it to the starting line. If running is something you want to continue doing after the initial event, and you maybe even want to go after some ambitious time goals, there are smarter ways to train that will both keep you healthy and make you a stronger runner. The less-is-more and weekend-warrior approaches will not give most of you the best results nor the most pleasant experiences, and this is true whether you are a novice or have been running for years.

I hate to be the bearer of bad news, but research does not support this approach. Don't get me wrong: there are many disagreements within the running and coaching community about what is best in training. If there was one agreed-upon approach, then everyone would be doing it. But things are not that simple. However, the fact remains that some approaches are clearly not as effective. While everyone has a right to their own opinion in all matters, not all opinions are equally sound—that is, not all opinions have adequate support needed to make them a reasonable claim. That's basic logic.

Returning to my favorite philosopher, Aristotle, he correctly notes that you can only seek the degree of precision that a subject allows: "Our discussion will be adequate if it has as much clearness as the subject matter admits of—for precision is not to be sought for alike in all discussions...look for precision in each class of things just so far as the nature of the subject admits—It is evidently equally foolish to accept probable reasoning from a mathematician and to demand from a rhetorician demonstrative proofs" (Barnes 1995). Take math: Math allows for precision. Two plus two equals four, and there's no disputing that. But empirical sciences are much more imprecise. And that's what we're dealing with here.

Training is messy business. We discover new things. Sometimes we need to adjust applications based on new findings. We must rely on the information we have, including research and experience—not our personal experience alone, which amounts to nothing more than hasty generalizations, though that may matter for us, but the whole of experience. There are at least three issues to consider here:

1. Aerobic and metabolic development
2. Training specificity
3. Running economy and efficiency

Aerobic and Metabolic Development

The only way to develop your aerobic and metabolic system for running long distances—and anything over 400 meters is primarily aerobic—is to run long distances, which serves to increase the number and size of mitochondria in your muscles. Mitochondria are the energy-producing factories in your body. Having more mitochondria means you can produce more energy for contracting muscles.

This means that weekly mileage matters, and the best way to get your necessary, and desirable, dose of mileage is with regular, fairly comfortable running. Easy running allows you to run more without getting injured or exhausted. Most runners run their easy runs too

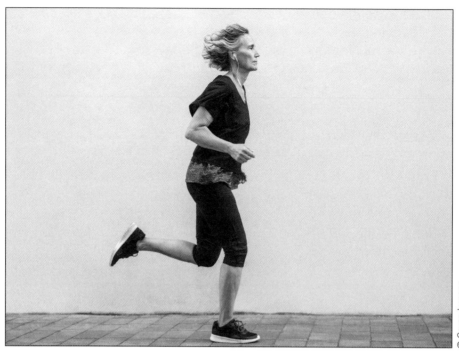

hard. There are several problems with running even just a bit too hard too often. First, you aren't training all the metabolic systems that need to be developed. Second, if you are always running just a bit too fast, you will likely be too tired to ever run really hard. For endurance training—and this does not apply to true sprint training—the combination of lots of easy miles plus some very hard running results in the greatest improvements. Running too fast too often neglects both sides of this equation (we'll talk more about this in a bit).

Now, let's say you take the less-is-more approach: One day you run hill repeats, one day you run intervals or a tempo run, then on the weekend you run long. If you only run a few quality hard runs a week, you are missing out on an essential part of your training. This approach is not optimal for developing a robust aerobic engine. Muscularly, you aren't training to optimize mitochondrial growth, and metabolically, you're not training your fatty acid fueling system. Basically, you're trying to build a house before you have a foundation on which to place your house.

The first step for any sort of training plan is to develop a wide base of aerobic capacity, upon which you can then build your speed. Easy and moderate running should make up 80 percent of your weekly mileage. Over time, this mileage serves many purposes:

- Endurance training increases and maximizes fat metabolism, improving the muscles' ability to oxidize (burn) fat for energy.

This adaptation means that the higher proportion of the energy needed for endurance exercise can come from fat rather than just carbohydrates or glycogen.

- Increases the number of aerobic enzymes, which are necessary for creating ATP, your primary energy source.
- Increases the size and number of mitochondria, which are the ATP factories of the cells, in your muscles.
- Increases capillarization, which delivers more oxygen and fuel and removes waste from muscles. Capillaries move blood into organs and tissues, bringing in oxygen and nutrients and removing waste products such as carbon dioxide.

Because these types of runs are relatively slow and long, lasting anywhere from 30 minutes to 3 hours, they get left out of the schedule in an aim to get more with less. They are often not viewed as quality runs, yet they are a necessary part of a well-developed system. And those doing the low-mileage, weekend-warrior approach just aren't getting enough of these miles. The result is that none of the previously listed critical adaptations can happen.

To illustrate this idea, consider the two triangles shown in figure 5.1. Optimal training for a goal event looks like a triangle, and the broader the base, the taller the peak can be. The narrower the base, the lower the peak, or the higher the likelihood that it may topple over. As you can see, the left triangle can still go much higher before it becomes unstable, while the one on the right is pretty maxed out at its current height. The deeper and broader your aerobic base, the higher your peak performance can be and the more likely you'll avoid injury because you've developed the physiological adaptations that allow your body to recover and absorb the training load. Once this base is developed, then you can add various types of speed workouts, which are necessary to build the peak toward your potential. But if the base is not there first, then the slightest ill wind will blow it over.

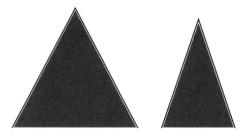

FIGURE 5.1 A broad base of aerobic conditioning allows for a high performance peak.

Training Specificity

A principle that applies to any sport, or any skill, is training specificity. If you want to become a good writer, you must write a lot. If you want to become a good artist, you must practice your craft a lot. If you want to master yoga, you must commit to your daily practice. If you want to be a good runner—and by "good," I mean able to do the things you want to do with running—you must run. Are there things you can do to help your running that are not running (like cross-training or strength work)? Yes. But those things should not replace running. They should be used to enhance and augment your running.

Additionally, when you're training for a goal, whatever that goal is, the training should become more specific to the demands of that particular goal as you get closer to the goal. If, for instance, you hope to run a strong 5K road race, you will focus on speed development as you get nearer to the race date.

But don't forget that distance running—anything longer than 400 meters or a few minutes of running—is primarily aerobic. Given that, specificity tells you that you should run as much as you can, given your individual body, time constraints, and goals. This comes first because it's the basis for any other desired adaptations.

Related to this is a very common myth deeply held by many runners: In order to run fast, you must train fast. This seems to be a reasonable assumption, and given my discussion earlier concerning specificity, it would seem obvious.

While this is true, it's often taken too far. This statement of fact is the number one piece of advice I hear from runners, whether they are a novice, intermediate, or experienced. They've heard it a million times, and they've bought into it lock, stock, and barrel. Why? It makes intuitive sense, and it's absolutely true. But the problem is that, as with many things in life, this isn't black and white. It's not an all-or-nothing proposition. If you're a sprinter racing 100 to 200 meters, then this is true. Sprinters need to run short distances at a very fast pace. But if you're running longer, then getting fast involves much more than just running fast, and that's because endurance events rely on a different type of muscle composition and fueling system.

Do you have to run fast to race fast? Yes, but not all the time. Fast running must be really fast and uncomfortable. Easy running must be comfortable and mostly pleasant. What I see time again with most runners, some of whom are quite experienced, is that all their runs are fairly fast, even for long runs. But they fail to run any of their runs fast enough.

What does it really matter if you run fast all the time? If you feel good, what's the harm? Shouldn't you be tuning in to how your body feels and run accordingly? You're always told, "Listen to your body!" Part of becoming a competent runner is learning how to sense where your body is and what it wants to do. There are two problems here: (1) It's all well and good to listen to your body, but it's actually very hard to shut your head out of the whole process. Are you really listening to your body? Is your brain, perhaps, whispering, "Come on. This is so slow. You'll feel better mentally if you pick it up a bit." (2) Your body doesn't know what's on tap for tomorrow. Perhaps your body joyfully proclaims, "Yay, I feel great! Let's run like the wind!" Your body doesn't know that you have a hard session planned for tomorrow—but you know that, don't you? There's a time to listen to your body and a time to tell it to shut up and listen to reason.

Let's suppose you have a hard workout scheduled for tomorrow, with long tempo, hills, and intervals, and today is an easy recovery run—but you wake up feeling fresh and springy. You have a busy day ahead of you and want to get moving, or perhaps you need to work out some stress from your soul and psyche. And so, instead of running your active recovery pace, you pound out some good heart-throbbing miles and return home pleasantly worked and ready to deal with your day. What's the harm in throwing in some extra fast running? How can that possibly hurt, especially when your body gives you unequivocal permission?

Well, this is the next question: Will you be able to get the same quality of run out of yourself tomorrow? With endurance training, both quality and quantity matter. You want to run enough miles, but the trick is to increase volume without sacrificing quality. And there's the rub. You cannot, over the course of weeks or months or years, increase volume and still have really high-quality hard runs if you do not respect the role of comfortable aerobic runs. At some point, you will either break down (from injury or deep fatigue), or you will plateau, or both.

> **With endurance training, both quality and quantity matter. You want to run enough miles, but the trick is to increase volume without sacrificing quality.**

Furthermore, aerobic running—at a pace you can carry on a conversation—taps into a different metabolic system. When you're running at a comfortable pace, you rely more on fat for fuel, sparing glycogen. If you run for 90 minutes or more, this system is crucial and really gets to work at this point. Running too fast means using more glycogen rather than fat, and so that metabolic system remains untrained.

The combination of slower aerobic runs and faster fast runs means you can maximize fat metabolism and lower the pace at which you continue to rely heavily on fat—your lactate threshold—sparing the limited glycogen you can store.

Lots of runners succumb to the notion that some miles are "junk miles," but those supposed junk miles are important if they're run correctly; otherwise, they're worse than junk. If you don't run them, you sacrifice volume (and all the benefits discussed earlier). Run them too fast, and you sacrifice quality. Run them just right, and you maximize your training for your present and future self. The only junk miles are miles that do nothing for you or that contribute to injury or stagnation.

Take the long view. Think not just of today, but of tomorrow. Think not just of tomorrow, but of next year, and the year after that. Running is a process. Developing the runner you can be is a state of becoming, not a state of being.

> **Running is a process. Developing the runner you can be is a state of becoming, not a state of being.**

Running Economy and Efficiency

While running may appear to be a simple movement, running efficiency will vary across individual runners. Running efficiency concerns how much energy you use per step. More efficient runners use less energy when running. Efficiency is affected by both running form and specific training. In both cases, runners become more efficient by running more. There are many ways to measure running efficiency or economy, such as the amount of oxygen consumed or the number of calories burned. Running efficiency has nothing to do with pace—you can be fast and efficient or slow and efficient.

Studies suggest that running form has very little to do with running efficiency. This may seem counterintuitive until you understand the complexity involved in a running gait (Patoz et al. 2022). Because running economy encompasses so many variables, chances are good that the way you're running is the most efficient for you. (There are a few form exceptions discussed in chapter 6).

However, the number one factor in improving running efficiency is running more. More mileage, more consistently, over months and years and decades will make you a more efficient runner. With most skills, you become more efficient at it the more you do it. This principle applies to running as well—both your movement and the cellular adaptations discussed earlier.

How to Build and Maintain a Robust Foundation

The previous section explains why it's good to build a deep aerobic base, but it doesn't explain how to do so. How do you start from zero?

How do you maintain an aerobic base while building on speed? How do you return from an injury or illness? How do you stay consistent? The first step is honestly assessing where you're at and where you want to go. If you're newer to running or if you believe there are areas you need to work on concerning some of the adaptations discussed earlier, here's the next question: How should you proceed?

Many adhere to what is commonly called the 10-percent rule. This rule states that a runner should not add more than 10 percent to their current training volume per week. Is the 10-percent rule actually a rule? Does it make sense, and does it work? Can you both build fitness and avoid injury using this rule? The answer is "yes" and "no" and "it depends."

Let's say you are currently running five miles a week, having recently started a couch-to-5K training plan. If you add 10 percent next week, that's half a mile. This is pretty minimal, and the truth is that you can probably add a mile or even two next week without any risk of injury. In terms of percentage, that's a big bump that would violate the 10-percent rule. But how you add that volume matters. If you run two miles three times a week and then add two miles to one of those runs, that may be pushing things. But let's say that instead, you add one mile to your longer run and a half mile to each of your other two runs. That's still a two-mile increase, but it spreads out the added stress while allowing you to benefit from the longer running. What's important here is to avoid adding too much to any single run.

Now let's say you're running 50 miles a week. Increasing next week's volume by 10 percent would take you to 55 miles. In this case, that's probably a safe addition. Again, you don't want to add that five miles to just one run.

Over time, this gradual increase in volume—keeping most of your running at a very comfortable pace, staying consistent, and adding in recovery weeks—will establish the aerobic foundation you need to add more goal-specific training. This also serves to strengthen your muscles, tendons, ligaments, and bones so that they, too, are prepared to handle higher demands. Once you have reached this point, however, you still need to maintain a strong base. This is not something you do once and then walk away and work on something else. If you're training for endurance, aerobic running must continue to make up the vast majority of your weekly miles, and then you can add in other types of runs, such as hill repeats, speed runs, progression runs, or downhill runs (you'll learn more about these later in the book). There are hundreds of variations possible (discussed in chapter 9).

Another important element in aerobic training, and training in general, is that you need to vary your runs, even when you're running at a similar effort level for most of your runs. What does that mean? It means that if you run five miles every day, you're limiting your improvement. Instead, make some runs a bit longer and some shorter. The longer days will be your harder days, and the shorter days are recovery days. If you want to start increasing one longer run, make sure it's balanced with your weekly volume. Your long run should not be more than 30 to 40 percent of your weekly total—so if you're running 20 miles a week, your long run would be about 7 miles, with the other 13 miles spread throughout the week. Too many runners make their longest run much too long, making them more susceptible to injury and sacrificing some very desirable adaptations.

In running, nothing can replace a solid aerobic base. Running lots of easy miles may not be sexy or exciting, but that consistency, discipline, and habit will reveal exciting new paths you never knew existed before. You may come to realize you can run a distance or a time that seemed inconceivable in the past. You may discover you can actually run without always being in pain. You may feel your strength and confidence improve as you witness yourself running more easily. You may start enjoying the very act of running as an end in itself, not simply a means to reach some goal, such as being healthier. Having a deep aerobic base will benefit every other running goal you have, and it will also make you feel better in your day-to-day life, now and for many years to come.

Chapter 6

Maximizing Training While Minimizing Injury

Many runners believe that cross-training is essential for staying healthy and injury-free. I would argue that cross-training can help in many cases—but it's not essential. The truth is, whether you're 30 or 60, or any age for that matter, you have your personal limits when it comes to how much running you can do and how much running you want to do. The principle of training specificity still rules if your goal is to become a better, stronger, faster runner: If you want to run better, you have to run. And with endurance running, the more you can run, the better. But there are lots of reasons to incorporate other activities that may either complement or support your primary goals.

While you may enjoy running, you may also enjoy other activities that enrich your life and recharge your mind and soul. Doing things you enjoy matters. Additionally, for some runners, running as much as they might like seems to lead to injuries. This could be due to doing too much, making some type of training mistake (such as running a bit too fast too often), or even accumulating injuries over the course of living. Whatever the reason, some wish to add cross-training into the mix. I will discuss the best options so that you can decide how best to fit these into your training based on your goals.

Cross-Train to Augment Running

This section is about the other types of training you can use to help build your running fitness for longevity and performance. You might be thinking, "This is a book for runners and about running." As I shared in chapter 5, in order to run well, you need to run. Running must be your primary activity if you want to be a runner and if you have running goals. If your goal is to include running in a general fitness program, then that changes the equation. The principle of specificity applies to everyone, no matter their age. But as you get older, adding in some cross-training and strength training can maximize your running and address some of the natural age-related muscle loss you face as time marches on.

> **Running must be your primary activity if you want to be a runner and if you have running goals.**

What does it mean to run as much as you can? Each one of you must find, over time and experimentation, where your training volume sweet spot is. Basically, over the course of your running life, you need to pay close attention to how your body responds to the training. This is the case whether you're 30 or 60. That never changes, but what you can handle when you're 30 may change by the time you're 60—or not. You see, what someone can handle concerning training volume—and here I'm really focusing on running volume—is relative to the individual.

Some runners can run 100 miles a week, but if they run 110 miles, they start to break down. Others can handle 30 miles a week, but running 35 doesn't feel good.

Part of this is the nature of training, and if you're still building a solid running base, then that 30 miles may just be your limit now and will increase gradually with smart, incremental changes. But if you've been running for years, you may have learned where your sweet spot is and that adding more only leads to trouble—either performance plateaus or injuries or both. One of the challenges is to find that point for yourself where running is a benefit. Once you find that, then you might look at adding in nonrunning training to improve your overall fitness.

Let me give you an example to help illustrate this approach: Let's say you've been running consistently for ten years. On average, you've maintained a weekly volume of 25 to 35 miles. Occasionally, you ramp this up a bit, but you find that if you go over 40 miles a week, you start feeling aches and pains that don't resolve after an easy day or two. You've noticed this happen a few times and now understand that your sweet spot is around 35 miles per week. That's what you can consistently run while recovering well. Now, you still want to increase your fitness, but you know that trying to run more will likely have the opposite result, so you consider adding cross-training while maintaining your 35-mile weeks. Of course, like anything, this cross-training needs to be added gradually.

What I'm suggesting is to use cross-training to augment, not replace, running. Cross-training can address weaknesses and increase training volume while avoiding additional impact that may increase injury risks. The options for cross-training are many and will depend on what you enjoy doing and what you have access to. Cross-training can also be used to enhance recovery, increase aerobic volume, and improve strength and mobility. Many activities qualify as cross-training. Here are some of the more common ones that runners use to augment their running:

Swimming and Other Water Exercise

Swimming, water aerobics, water running, and other water exercises can be used to increase training volume and improve joint mobility, core strength, and recovery time. Full disclosure—I encourage every runner to swim. You can derive so much benefit from swimming because it:

- *Increases ankle and foot mobility.* Swimming encourages plantar flexion (where your toes are pointed away from your body), while running is a very dorsiflexion-dominant activity.

- *Improves cardiorespiratory fitness through breath control.* Because swimming involves holding your breath, and breathing is dictated by arm strokes, it forces your body to use the oxygen it has.
- *Incorporates core muscles and increases arm-swing power and arm mobility.* Since good running dynamics rely on a strong core and rotational force, this will make you a stronger runner.
- *Improves cardiac fitness.* You can add aerobic work without additional impact stress. With running, you are often walking a fine line between doing too much and doing just the right amount. Adding water activities can help you manage this balance while improving cardiorespiratory fitness.
- *Incorporates resistance training.* Water is 800 percent denser than air, so exercise in water counts as resistance training. Water jogging allows a runner to recover from injury or add exercise volume that's still quite specific to running, again without the added impact.
- *Improves recovery in a non-weight-bearing manner.* Research suggests that swimming for recovery enhances exercise performance the following day compared to passive recovery (a nonactive rest day). It also appears that swimming lowers muscle inflammation (Lum, Landers, and Peeling 2010).
- *Reduces the risk of injury.* Swimming allows you to add more training or to replace some running with low-impact activity.

The last two points are important because many runners are reluctant to give up a run on their schedule even when they feel something concerning going on—a little tweak that isn't going away or muscle soreness that's been hanging on for several days. Swimming lets you take that day off and allow your body extra time to heal while still getting a workout in. As you will learn in chapter 7, recovery is a priority if you want to continue to run.

You can swim after a run to increase your training volume. Because swimming introduces the lowest biomechanical stress compared to the other cross-training options, it allows you to safely increase training load without increasing injury risk.

Cycling

Cycling—road, gravel, indoor, or mountain—can be used as recovery if you're taking a short, comfortable ride. Or you can throw in a hard spin class, long road ride, or hilly mountain-bike ride to add some quality training without the pounding of running. You can also add a short ride after a run to increase overall volume without the same risk of injury.

While cycling works different muscles than running does, this can complement running by balancing out muscle imbalances. An easy ride moves healing blood through your muscles, which helps recovery. If you're feeling muscle aches, replacing an easy recovery run with an easy aerobic spin can allow you added recovery while maintaining training load.

Rowing

Lots of people believe that rowing is primarily for the upper body, but it's really a leg-driven activity. It also involves your core, and that will benefit your running and overall fitness and make you less prone to injury. Like other low-impact exercises, rowing provides an excellent cardiorespiratory workout without added impact. While rowing engages the leg muscles, it also strengthens the core, back, arms, and shoulders, which can help with running posture and resistance training.

Elliptical

The elliptical closely mimics a running motion, so I usually recommend this for runners who feel they can't increase their running due to impact-related soreness and those who are building their running base and want to alternate days of running with running-specific cross-training. Because the elliptical is more specific to running but does not have the same high-impact forces, it's very useful for those who are newer to running and don't want the pounding of running every day or those who just need to balance the stresses of running while keeping their training load steady.

Strength Training

For older runners, I do not consider strength training to be cross-training in the traditional sense of offering different activities that mimic or balance out running. Cross-training is not essential for good running. You can train for running without any cross-training. However, while it may offer you some other options and you may reap some training benefits, I don't see strength training as optional, at least for runners 50 and over. Strength training is crucial to counteract the natural process of muscle mass and strength loss. As you get older, running is no longer enough to maintain muscle.

There's lots of debate concerning what type of strength training is best, such as high repetitions and low weight versus low repetitions and high weight. My feeling is that both are beneficial for different reasons, but ultimately, it's heavy lifting that will offer more bang for the buck. Heavy lifting recruits all the muscle fibers and demands joint stabilization. Also, as you get older, your anabolic hormones decrease. Heavy lifting makes the most of what you have. For women in particular, who experience a sharp drop in estrogen, heavy lifting maximizes the estrogen you do have.

Heavy lifting is also good for your bones, not just your muscles. Bone, like all other tissues in the body, only maintains the strength it needs. Demand determines strength. Bones that are stressed, but not overstressed, remain strong. Remove the stress, and bones no longer maintain their density and strength. Like with muscles, tendons, and ligaments, you either use them or lose them. Bones require force to remain strong. This means that muscles must pull on them—forcefully. While body-weight impact activities like walking and running can help, heavy lifting is even better for bones because the force is greater.

There's one important caveat concerning heavy lifting: You must lift correctly. Form matters, and there's really no wiggle room on this. Lifting using poor form is much worse than not lifting at all. As a NASM-certified personal trainer, I recommend doing several sessions with a trainer who is experienced working with older athletes or female athletes (if that applies to you). They will take you through a developmental progression based on your current fitness level. Starting off with too many weighted squats or lunges when you have not mastered the mechanics is a recipe for injury.

There are seven fundamental movement patterns that should all be incorporated into your strength training. Let's look at each one.

Pull

Pulling exercises involve contracting muscles to bring a resistance toward your body. Most pull exercises target the back, biceps, and forearms, but exercises such as hamstring curls are also pull exercises. Other examples of pull exercises are pull-ups, chin-ups, lat pull-downs, bent-over rows, bicep curls, and hamstring curls.

Press or Push

Press or push exercises involve extending your arms against a resistance and moving the resistance away from your body. Examples of press or push exercises are push-ups, bench presses, overhead presses, shoulder presses, dumbbell chest presses, dips, and leg presses.

Carry

Carry exercises involve holding a weight and walking with it. These are very beneficial functional exercises. Examples of carry exercises include the farmer's carry, suitcase carry, and sandbag carry.

Lunge

Lunges involve stepping forward, backward, or sideways and bending at the knees with an upright torso. They are similar to squats but are a bit more balanced and knee-dominant. You can do these with or without weight.

Squat

Squats involve bending at the knees and hips while keeping your torso upright. Squats primarily strengthen the quadriceps, hamstrings, and glutes. Squatting exercises include front squats, back squats, goblet squats, and overhead squats. Bulgarian split squats are a variation of single-leg squats. Because running is a one-legged action, Bulgarian split squats are very beneficial for runners.

Rotation

Rotational movements involve twisting your limbs and torso around the center axis of the body. While many activities are either frontal or lateral, running actually involves all planes, since the movement between the upper body and lower body involves a rotation that helps to move you forward. Rotational exercises involve both the rotation and the control (antirotation) of that rotation. Examples of rotational exercises are medicine ball throws and woodchoppers; antirotational exercises include dead bug, bird dog plank pull-throughs, and single-leg deadlifts.

Hinge

Hinge movements are lower-body movements that involve bending at the hips while maintaining a straight spine. Hinge movements target the posterior chain, including the hamstrings, glutes, and lower back. These are the muscles that move you in a forward direction. With hinges, the knees are soft with a slight bend, but the main action is at the hips. Examples of hinge exercises are bridges, hip thrusts, deadlifts, Romanian deadlifts, and kettlebell swings.

Mobility Work

Mobility work focuses on your joints and the surrounding muscles. Mobility is about the movement of your joints and your range of motion (ROM). Warming up before a run with a short mobility routine allows your body to move more fluidly, reducing the chance of injury and allowing you to run more comfortably. This is something you can easily add before each run. Just a few minutes will reap major benefits.

Let's look at a typical application: Perhaps you've been sitting at your desk all day at work. You're getting ready for your evening run. Sitting all day has allowed your hip flexors, the front and top of your legs where they meet your torso, to shorten and tighten (overactivation). Meanwhile, your backside has been overstretched all day (underactivation). And your hips—oh, your hips just ache. But you get dressed and trot off on your run, feeling as creaky as the Tin Man in *The Wizard of Oz*. You hobble down the road with reduced ROM, which makes you more susceptible to injury and undermines your performance.

Instead, try a few dynamic body-weight mobility exercises to warm up. Add some walking lunges with upper body rotation, side lunges, skips, mountain climbers, butt kicks, karaoke exercises or crossovers, or leg swings. Your muscles, tendons, and ligaments will be warmed up, and your ROM will allow you to run more comfortably and safely. Mobility work can be added at other times as well, just to improve your overall ROM. This can be done with myofascial release, dynamic stretching, and body-weight strength work.

Some strength work also serves as mobility work, such as lunges, single-leg deadlifts, squats, bridges, and kettlebell swings. The dynamic warm-up exercises provided in chapter 8 also target ROM. Add in hurdle steps (forward and backward), ankle circles (clockwise and counterclockwise), and leg swings (forward, backward, and side-to-side), and you'll hit the key areas that will keep your body feeling flexible and fluid.

Concerning all the previous suggestions, it's important to keep in mind that you must always add things slowly and remember the principle that hard days should be hard and easy days should be easy. Lifting hard on a running recovery day does not make that a recovery day. As I discuss in chapter 7, stress is stress—the body cannot differentiate between running stress, lifting stress, biking stress, or life stress. Pay attention to all of these. Some days need to be very easy, and just because you're doing something different doesn't mean it's easy. Debilitating fatigue, injury, and diminishing returns will be the result if you try to push it hard every day, even if you're pushing it hard in different ways. Respect recovery.

Use Proper Running Technique

Several years ago, running technique became the big subject of discussion and debate in running. Some of it has merit, and some of it does not. But one of the important things I've learned as I've studied this closely is that every runner has a unique running gait. Your running gait is the result of a lot of things going on with your individual body, and what may work for you may not work for another person.

The classic case is the contentious debate concerning foot strike—how your foot lands on impact at midstance. Is it bad to heel strike? Is it good to run on your forefoot? Is a midfoot strike better? Since this discussion began, I've learned a lot thanks to research. Of course, all this is bound to change, but right now, I have some understanding of what likely does and does not matter concerning running gait.

So, is heel striking bad? No, unless you are overstriding. Overstriding is when your foot is ahead of your center of mass on impact, meaning your foot lands ahead of your body. If you land on your heel and your foot is under your body when you land, then that's fine. A midfoot strike is also fine. Landing on your forefoot is fine too, but unless you're a sprinter running 100 meters, running *only* on your forefoot will stress your posterior chain and likely cause calf and Achilles issues.

> **Your** running gait is the result of a lot of things going on with your individual body, and what may work for you may not work for another person.

Then there is the issue of cadence: the number of steps you take per minute. Cadence is important to address if it is very low. Many say the ideal cadence is 180 steps per minute. But as with most things, there is a range, and it will depend a bit on your body. A cadence of 180, plus or minus 10, is reasonable (so that means 170 to 190 is fine). If you are below or above, then that's something to look at. If you have either a very low or very high cadence, efficiency is the concern. With a very low cadence, the increased ground time (the time your foot is on the ground) can increase injury risks.

Regarding other form concerns, be careful about what you adjust. Yes, you want to run upright, eyes focused ahead and not on your feet, arms relaxed and crossing to the midline of your body, jaw relaxed (this is the key to a relaxed body), and steps quiet. But getting too caught up in some idea of an ideal running gait is misguided. Note: some of the best runners ever have had running gaits that are almost painful to watch. That does not mean they couldn't have benefited from a more efficient gait, but it's important to recognize that your running gait is very individual. Some things can and should be addressed, such as overstriding or very low cadence, and other things just reflect your unique body.

Running Shoe Considerations

This is the number one question I hear from runners: "What's the best running shoe?" My answer is always that there is no best shoe. There is the best shoe for *you*, but not an objectively best shoe in general. The one thing you must understand about shoes is that they should feel good on your feet. Running shoes must fit the shape of your foot and allow adequate toe and forefoot spread on impact. It doesn't matter what shoes are advertised as the best or fastest or most cushioned.

(continued)

Running Shoe Considerations *(continued)*

It doesn't matter what shoes your friend loves, and it doesn't matter what color they are. All that matters is that they feel good when you put them on your feet and while running.

Running shoes are the most important piece of equipment a runner needs. If possible, do not skimp on running shoes. In running shoes, you usually get what you pay for, so those bargain knockoffs may feel okay for a few weeks, but they will likely break down much faster than a high-end shoe. In the end, you'll pay more, both for new shoes and perhaps for treating injuries that you could have avoided.

Anatomy of a Running Shoe

When you shop for running shoes, it's helpful to understand how they are put together and what that means for supporting you. Let's take a look:

- *Soles:* The outersole is the material on the bottom of the shoe that hits the ground, while the midsole is the material between the outersole and the upper of the shoe, which holds your foot. The insole lies inside the shoe for added cushion and comfort. Insoles can also be changed to suit individual needs, such as additional arch support.

- *Drop:* A shoe's drop refers to the difference in midsole thickness between the front and back of the shoe. Shoes generally have drops anywhere from 0 to 12 millimeters. There are a lot of theories about what drop is best, but keep in mind that different shoes work for different runners. The options are there because different runners like different shoes.

- *Stack:* A shoe's stack refers to the overall height of the shoe—how much material is between you and the ground. This mostly concerns cushioning; a higher-stack shoe normally comes with more cushioning. A lower-stack shoe generally has less cushioning, and you can feel the ground more under your feet. More cushioning is not always a good thing, though, because it also introduces instability—by allowing more movement in your foot, ankle, and leg—and proprioceptive difficulties. As each foot lands, millions of nerves in your feet send signals to your brain telling your body where you are in space. Highly cushioned shoes can make this more difficult. For some, highly cushioned shoes may feel good on the foot but may cause issues higher up the kinetic chain, often in the knees, hips, and lower back.

Types of Running Shoes

Based on your preferences and needs, you'll likely have many options for shoes. An experienced salesperson at a running-shoe store may also be able to guide you toward the shoe that has the optimal features for you. Let's take a look:

- *Neutral shoes:* These do not provide medial support but do provide some degree of cushion and protection. For the most part, they allow your feet to move naturally without external control.
- *Stability shoes:* Stability shoes provide varying degrees of medial support for runners who pronate too much. Pronation is a natural movement of the foot where the foot rolls inward during the ground-contact phase of the stride. Pronation is part of your natural shock-absorption system. But if you roll inward too much, this can place excessive stress on your ankles, knees, and on up your body (the kinetic chain). Overpronation can be caused by a biomechanical issue, foot weakness, or even hip or core weakness. It is always better to strengthen the system than to add external support for a weakness. Any added external support will only further weaken the system. Remember, your body only maintains the strength you need. Bodies are very efficient at not doing what they don't have to do.
- *Trail shoes:* As the name suggests, these are specifically made for running on trails. They usually have a more aggressive outsole for traction, and they are just a bit more stable on uneven surfaces. Some also have rock plates that protect your feet from sharp rocks and roots.
- *Minimal shoes:* These shoes provide minimal support and cushioning. They allow for natural foot movement and ground feel.
- *Maximal shoes:* By contrast, these shoes provide substantial cushioning.

Now that you know the terms, you can go to your local running store and find the shoe that's right for you. Studies show that most people buy shoes based on aesthetics, especially color. While that may be understandable, it's the least important attribute for a running shoe. Remember, shoes are important for safety and enjoyment while you run. Choose wisely.

Be Aware of Common Running Injuries

Productive training requires a balance of building up miles and strengthening your body. Overloading or underloading your system can result in either injury or fitness plateaus. Many believe that injuries are a necessary part of running. I'm generally not one of those people, but when you do things that push your limits, you do place yourself at risk for these things.

There are two types of injuries common in running: acute and chronic. Acute injuries include an ankle roll, a bad fall that injures your knee or some other body part, or a sudden muscle tear. Generally, this covers things that happen suddenly and are not specifically due to training. Chronic, or overuse, injuries are due to the stress you impose on your body day in and day out. They tend to happen slowly over time and can be a bit insidious. You may feel something not quite right and think, "Should I run or rest this?" The stresses placed on your body gradually compromise structures over time and lead to injuries such as tendinitis, stress fractures, strained ligaments, joint issues, and pain caused by tight fascia. These overuse injuries are avoidable with proper training. The acute injuries are more difficult to avoid because accidents happen, but in some cases, weak underlying structures can contribute to those accidents. A fall could be due to chronic stress and poor recovery, leading to limited mobility and muscular imbalances. That hamstring pull might not have come out of nowhere; maybe you've been feeling a little extra tightness recently.

One thing to consider as you continue your running journey is to have a good physical therapist (PT) on your team. Look for someone who has experience working with runners and practices a variety of modalities such as Astym, e-stim, ultrasound, cold laser, dry needling, and Graston Technique. Many of these modalities will help treat soft-tissue irritations or tightness, restore movement, and reduce pain. It's beneficial to catch any burgeoning issues early, and having access to a good PT you trust and who is familiar with you can really help you avoid lingering issues.

Before discussing specific issues, I want to offer some general guidelines when dealing with different types of injuries. Most overuse injuries concern tendon or ligament stress. Tendons and ligaments need blood to heal. Unfortunately, they do not naturally receive a lot of blood. Inflammation is your body's response to injury and stress; it's a healing response. Many falsely believe that all inflammation is bad and must be reduced. Too much inflammation is not good, but some inflammation *is* good. In the case of tendon and ligament overuse injuries, inflammation helps bring healing blood to the affected area. Using ice and anti-inflammatory medications undermines this natural healing process. Muscle strains can benefit from ice initially if there is a good amount of swelling. In the case of muscles, excessive swelling can further damage the tissue.

So, here's a general rule, and of course rules always have some exceptions, but: For muscle strains or tears, ice and anti-inflammatories are good initially to get the swelling down. For tendon and ligament injuries, heat is best. In all cases, you do not want to stretch injured tissue. Light rolling and self-massage can help, but stretching will most likely only further stress the already-compromised tissue. Stretching may be prescribed during recovery and rehab, but not during the healing process.

While it's outside the scope of this book to cover every possible injury or offer treatment protocols, I'll discuss the more common ones here. You may have experienced some of these in the past if you've been running for many years, or these may be new to you either because you're relatively new to running or because your body responds to running differently as you get older. Either way, be aware of how these injuries may be caused and what to look for so you can identify them quickly and take action to prevent them from becoming issues that keep you from running.

Shin Splints

Medial tibial stress syndrome (MTSS), also known as shin splints (see figure 6.1), is felt on the front inner shin along the tibia, or shinbone. The pain here can be caused by several issues concerning the muscles and tendons along the front of your lower leg, and the pain can travel down to your ankles and feet. It's important to know that this injury involves muscle, tendon, and bone. This pain can also be associated with a stress fracture or stress reaction, so ruling that out first is important. If left untreated, MTSS can lead to a tibial stress fracture.

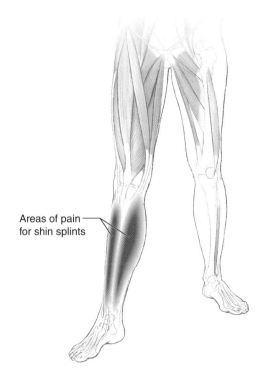

FIGURE 6.1 Shin splints.

There are several possible causes for shin splints:

- *Training error:* A sudden increase in training load may not allow your body enough time to adapt. Adding more demands than your body can handle too quickly will lead to muscle, tendon, and ligament injuries. Progressive overload allows you to gradually increase demands on your body that your body can handle. Pain is caused by stress that either your bones or your connective tissues are not yet equipped to handle.
- *Biomechanics:* If your feet pronate excessively, that places additional stress on the medial side of the shin. This pronation may be due to foot weakness or even hip or core weakness.
- *Footwear:* Sometimes, changing to a very different type of running shoe or running in broken-down shoes can add uneven stresses. For example, if you pronate a bit but are running in worn-out shoes where the medial midsole has broken down, this leads to additional inward roll. Likewise, switching to a shoe that is quite different from the shoe you have been running in may introduce new movement patterns that your body needs to adjust to—switching from a stabilizing shoe to a neutral shoe, for example. You should gradually work the new shoe into your rotation rather than wearing it for every run as soon as you get it.

Many runners believe that shin splints are caused by running on hard surfaces, but this is not the case. Shin splints are caused by adding too much mileage or speed—or both—too quickly, which stresses not only the muscles and tendons along the bone but also the bone itself. When bone is not given enough time to adapt and remodel, pain results. Those who most commonly deal with MTSS are newer runners and athletes returning to running after a break. The pain is the product of applying too much stress to the bone when it has not built the necessary strength.

MTSS is a sign that you need to pull things back and rest to allow time for adaptation. Pushing through this type of injury will make matters worse; it's not something you can just keep running through. Running on soft surfaces and in cushioned shoes may sound like a logical step, but research has shown that running on softer surfaces actually increases leg stiffness to compensate. Running on soft surfaces also presents proprioceptive challenges. Each time your foot hits the ground, millions of nerve endings in the foot sense where you are in space and send signals to your brain telling your body how to adjust. Landing on a soft surface makes this more challenging because each step is unstable.

Plantar Fasciitis

Plantar fasciitis (PF) usually presents as pain in the arch of the foot, often near the heel or just inside the heel, closer to the ankle (see figure 6.2). The first sign of a problem is often stiffness and pain when first getting out of bed in the morning or after sitting for a long period of time. Once you start walking around, the ligament warms and loosens, and the pain subsides. But if it's not addressed, it will progress, making even walking painful.

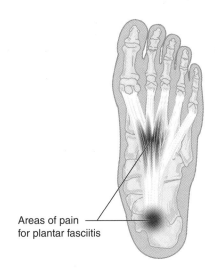

FIGURE 6.2 Plantar fasciitis.

There are many possible causes of PF. The most likely culprits are weak feet, tight calves, or an underactive gluteus medius. Other injuries can present similarly, such as tibialis posterior tendinitis and Baxter's nerve entrapment (less common but still something to be aware of). If you're not sure what you're dealing with, see a PT for an assessment.

Many runners ask, "Can I run with PF?" The answer is yes and no. With this injury, it's very important to tune in to the signals your body is sending you. If you can run fairly pain-free after a short, easy warm-up, then yes, you can continue running, but you need to back off the speed and keep things as flat as possible. If you're running on roads, make sure they are not excessively cambered (sloped toward the outsides of the road), especially if that causes your injured foot to roll more inward. Activity is generally helpful for healing injured ligaments and tendons. Neither ligaments nor tendons have good blood supplies, but they need the nutrients that blood brings in to be able to heal. Moderate activity helps with this and has been shown to aid in healing more than complete rest. But it's a balance, and you need to listen to what your body is telling you. Heat is also beneficial for ligament and tendon overuse injuries.

However, if the pain does not back off after a warm-up, and if it's compromising your normal running gait, it's a good idea to seek out cross-training options such as biking or swimming. See a PT if it doesn't get better.

Runner's Knee

Runner's knee is a common name for generalized knee pain, clinically described as patellofemoral pain syndrome (see figure 6.3). It is most often felt as a dull pain under or below the kneecap, but it can also present as a grinding or cracking below the kneecap. It can cause pain going down stairs, sitting down or standing up from a seated position, squatting, or kneeling.

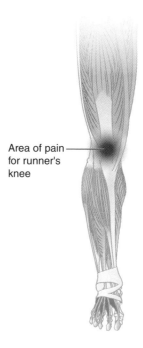

FIGURE 6.3 Runner's knee.

Runner's knee can be caused by overtraining (doing too much too soon), which often causes pain just below the kneecap due to an overworked patella tendon, or tracking issues sometimes brought on by muscle imbalances or weaknesses. Strengthening your quads, hips, and glutes—plus rolling your quads—while backing off on running can help resolve this. Adding in cycling to strengthen your quads and swimming to help maintain your training load without exacerbating the issues causing the injury can help you recover, get stronger, and avoid ongoing issues.

Achilles Tendinitis or Tendinopathy

Achilles tendons are the strongest and largest in the body. As is the case with all tendons, they function like springs. Energy is stored in them on impact and released at takeoff. Healthy tendons are not soft. Tendons are made up of collagen fibers all laid closely together in parallel. When tendons are damaged, the collagen fibers begin to separate, and the parallel structure starts to break down. Instead of a neat pattern of parallel fibers, you have collagen fibers resembling a bowl of spaghetti, resulting in a soft tendon that cannot withstand the strains placed on it. This injury process is the same for all tendinitis or tendinopathy.

When you run, the load applied to the Achilles tendon is around three times your body weight. Over the course of a run, that adds up to a lot of stress. Any of the following can cause extra stress if your body isn't trained to manage it:

- Fast or explosive running or other activities
- Downhill running
- High-volume running
- Running at a high intensity
- Tight calf muscles
- Excessive pronation
- Transitioning to low-drop shoes too quickly
- Anything that results in a dramatic load increase on the tendon

There are two types of Achilles tendinitis (see figure 6.4):

1. *Insertional tendinitis:* This is felt at the heel and is a compression injury.
2. *Midpoint Achilles tendinitis:* Pain is felt higher up the tendon. Sometimes the tendon will feel tender when pinched, there might be a lump somewhere along the tendon, or you might feel a subtle grinding (crepitation) when pinching the tendon and flexing and relaxing it.

The trick with Achilles tendinitis is that every case is different. For some runners, continuing moderate training may be feasible. For others, that will make matters worse. In every case, you must pay close attention to how your Achilles feels during and after activity.

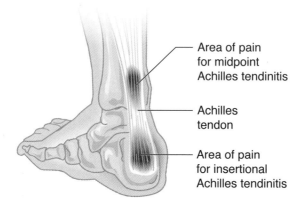

FIGURE 6.4 Achilles tendinitis: insertional and midpoint.

Catching this injury early is very important. When caught early, you can often fix it with a short reduction in training volume and intensity. But identifying the cause is crucial to avoid a flare-up. Many runners get caught in a cycle of injury, recovery, rebuild, and reinjury because they fail to identify the cause. Consult with a PT if your attempts to recover are not working.

Iliotibial Band Syndrome

Iliotibial band syndrome, or ITB syndrome, most often presents as pain just superior to (above) the lateral side of the knee (see figure 6.5). The ITB is made of thick fascia that provides stability from your pelvis down to your knee. It attaches at the top of your pelvis and inserts at the outside of your knee. There are several important muscles that attach to this fascia, including the gluteus medius, gluteus maximus, tensor fasciae latae (TFL), lateral quadricep, and lateral hamstring. At the attachment and insertion points, where the ITB is attached to bone, there's a fat pad and bursa for cushioning.

Fascia does not stretch. Its purpose is to provide support and tension. It used to be believed that ITB syndrome was a friction injury caused by the tissue moving over bone at the attachment or insertion point. But current research suggests that ITB syndrome is likely caused by excessive compression of the fat pad or bursa. Too much tension on the fascia—often caused by muscle weaknesses and imbalances (such as glute weakness or an overly active, shortened, or tight TFL), running on a cambered road, running with a leg-length discrepancy, adding a lot of downhill running too quickly, or excessive foot pronation—presses on the fat pad and bursa, causing trauma and inflammation.

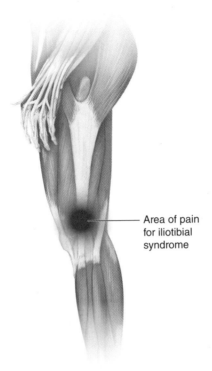

FIGURE 6.5 Iliotibial band syndrome.

While stretching may help, it's the muscles attached to the fascia band that should be stretched, not the fascia—because it will not stretch. Many recommend foam rolling, but again, it's the muscles around the band that should be rolled, not the fascia itself. Depending on pain level, you may be able to continue running as you add specific strength work and, ideally, physical therapy.

Stress Fractures

Stress fractures are tiny cracks in the bone caused by repeated stress that is just a bit beyond what the bone can handle (see figure 6.6). Bones, like any other part of the body, will break when subjected to more force than they can tolerate. Many view bones as static objects, but just as tendons, ligaments, and muscles grow stronger over time in response to stress, so, too, do bones. The only caveat here is that it's harder to strengthen bones later in life.

Peak bone density is reached in your early 30s. Building bone strength after 50 is more difficult but still possible. The best way to increase bone strength is to place heavy loads on the bone; you need to do things that cause your muscles to exert strong force on the ends of

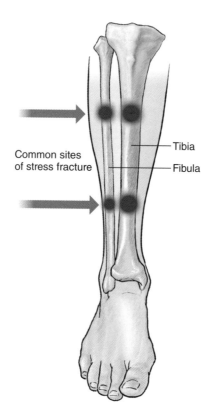

FIGURE 6.6 Stress fracture.

the bone. Heavy strength work, which means low repetitions and heavy weight, is the most effective. However, this needs to be progressive and gradual. While impact activity, such as running, is good for your bones, running alone will not build bone strength.

You cannot run through a stress fracture—ever. Unlike connective tissue, bone healing is a bit more predictable, but in order for a stress fracture to heal, you must rest the injury. If you continue to run on it or participate in activities that stress the bone, you may end up with a much more serious bone break with a longer recovery.

Hamstring Strain

A hamstring strain is felt in the belly of the hamstring muscles that run down the back of your thigh (see figure 6.7). Severe strains and tears are quite rare in distance running, but for those who focus on sprinting and more explosive running, this can be an issue. Mild strains are not uncommon and are a result of—you guessed it—overdoing something.

Inadequate warm-ups, overly tight quadriceps, and weak glutes can lead to hamstring strains. Again, this is an injury you want to

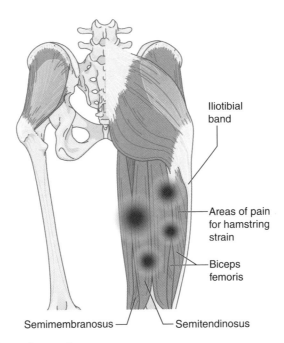

FIGURE 6.7 Hamstring strain.

address quickly. Since it's a muscle injury, ice and rest can be helpful initially. In most cases, a nonacute hamstring injury—one that comes on slowly not due to an explosive movement—suggests that specific strengthening is needed once the pain calms down.

Proximal Hamstring Tendinopathy

Proximal hamstring tendinopathy presents as pain at the sit bone and is much more common in endurance running (see figure 6.8). This is an injury to the tendon where the hamstring attaches to the base of the pelvis. The causes include the following:

- *Sitting:* Too much sitting or sitting on hard surfaces can cause a compression injury.
- *Training mistakes:* Too much hill running or sprinting added too quickly can injure the tendon.
- *Stretching:* Stretching too much or too far or stretching once you start feeling pain will make this injury worse.

When treating proximal hamstring tendinopathy, the following actions may help:

- Reduce the compression (don't sit too much or too long, or sit on a soft surface)

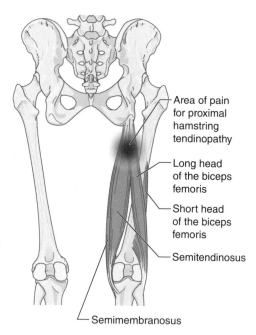

FIGURE 6.8 Proximal hamstring tendinopathy.

- Apply heat
- Add light foam rolling and massage of the hamstring muscle
- Avoid stretching
- Increase your foot turnover (cadence) to shorten your stride and reduce stress
- Take a break from speed and hill work

This is an injury that most can run through, but it compromises your running. As I've already noted, tendon injuries do benefit from blood-moving activity, but too much will cause this injury to linger.

It is beyond the scope of this book to detail all common running injuries, but the most important piece of advice I will offer is this: Listen to your body. Your body knows what's going on. It's very smart. My second piece of advice is to have some professionals on your team: Find a PT you trust. Add a massage therapist, a chiropractor, a personal trainer, and maybe even a running coach. Having a team behind you when you hit a bump in the road can keep you healthy. Having trusted professionals to turn to when you feel something may need attention will help you avoid serious injuries that can lead to long downtimes.

There's nothing better for your running than staying healthy and consistent. Catching things early, recognizing that something may be a problem, and nipping potential issues in the bud allows for the consistency that is key to staying in the game. The repeated training interruptions that injuries cause can undermine your well-being—physically, mentally, emotionally, and socially. And as you get older, long layoffs are more difficult to come back from. Set yourself up now for those times when something doesn't feel quite right. Take care of your amazing body that will take you to amazing places for years to come.

As we get older, there are certain things that we need to pay more attention to, specifically recovery and strength work, but we can continue to train for the things we wish to do, whether that's running daily, pursuing ambitious race goal, or wherever your dreams and desires lead you.

Chapter 7

Incorporating Rest and Recovery

I've said this several times, but let me repeat it: Stress plus recovery equals increased strength. Getting stronger means many things in this case. You can run farther, faster, more often, more comfortably, injury-free, and for a lifetime, if that's your goal. You feel better and more energetic throughout your day. You remain vibrant and active and able to pursue the activities you want to continue doing. To do all that, recovery must be an integral part of your plan.

As mentioned before, what many runners fail to recognize is that recovery isn't the absence of training—recovery *is* training. Recovery is as necessary as any other workout. Runners commonly have a hard time truly embracing real rest and recovery because they often believe fitness is lost when they are either resting (no workout) or taking an easy recovery day (light activity). The balance of stress and recovery is not always easy to find, but it's important to understand that training stress, just like any stress, if it is chronic and greater than you can adapt to, undermines your well-being and progress.

The Need for Rest and Recovery

Recovery is part of any good training plan, but as you get older, recovery tends to be even more important. Many find that they recover more slowly as they age. So, the challenge is to recover well and do everything you can to improve recovery time. Many runners succumb to the idea that if they just keep working harder, they'll perform better. You may think that if one hard workout isn't bringing down your times or allowing you to run farther, then you'd better add more work; maybe you just need to work harder. But does this approach really work? In reality, the benefit of a particular run or any other workout is both the work—which will result in muscular microtears, metabolic responses, and other reactions—and the recovery that allows stressed muscles, tendons, ligaments and metabolic, endocrine, and nervous systems to heal and become stronger in the process. If that healing does not happen, you will only get weaker, slower, and more susceptible to injury. Often, you must work smarter, not harder.

Recovery periods are a part of every phase of training: macrocycle, mesocycle, and microcycle. You can plan recovery weekly, semiregularly during a training cycle (such as every fourth week), annually (substantially cut back on volume and intensity for a week to several weeks), or even based on how you are responding to the training you're doing.

Here are some signs that recovery is needed, even when it's not on the schedule:

- Elevated resting heart rate for a few days
- Elevated heart rate during normal daily activities or during runs

- Sleep disturbances
- Irritability
- The feeling that your effort is greater while your paces are slowing
- Ongoing muscle soreness that does not improve following a rest or recovery day

Scheduling regular recovery days, weeks, and even months can prevent injuries, burnout, and performance plateaus. And being willing to add recovery time when needed is the key to healthy running.

There are some situations where recovery is standard practice. Take, for example, the end of a training cycle, or macrocycle. Suppose you've just run a goal race or reached some other personal running or fitness goal. How should you approach the next week or month? The answer depends on the demands placed on you in reaching that goal. If you just trained for your first marathon or completed your first couch-to-5K program, you may need more recovery than if you've been through this many times before. There's a standard recommendation that for every mile you race, you should allow one day for recovery. However, if you just ran your first 10K, and you ran it at a very hard effort, you'll likely need more than six days to really feel recovered. Likewise, if you just ran your 100th marathon, you probably won't need 26 days to recover. But this is all very individual, so you must learn to listen to your body and understand what it's telling you.

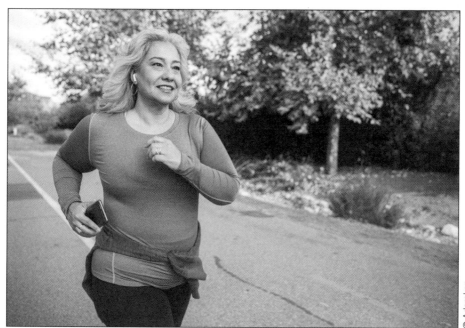

© Adamkaz

It's important to understand that there are physiological impacts of racing that you may not immediately feel. As an example, studies show that after a marathon, certain cardiac inflammation markers are elevated. You may not feel this, but it's there. Likewise, there are also muscular microtears that need time to heal. Respect the recovery, even if you feel like you don't need to recover.

Recovery Protocols

The recovery business has grown in recent years, but some protocols work better than others, and some can even undermine your recovery. Let's take a look at some of the more popular protocols used in recovery today.

Postrun Nutrition

There is a postworkout window of maximum carbohydrate absorption, allowing you to restock your glycogen supply quickly and effectively. Studies indicate that this window lasts between 30 and 60 minutes after a workout. This glycogen will be there for your next run or workout. You should aim for a three-to-one ratio of carbohydrates to protein (Murray and Rosenbloom 2018). While many look for elusive ergogenic aids—special supplements or vitamins to help you recover faster, feel better and less achy overall, look younger, and move more fluidly—what you don't see is that your diet plays a major role in how you feel as you age. Merely adding a light recovery drink, which can be as simple as a glass of chocolate milk (containing carbohydrates and protein) or a formulated recovery drink, after more a demanding exercise helps jump-start the healing process and reloads your working tissues for the rest of the day and the next day. Since recovery times for older runners are generally longer, this postrun nutrition boost becomes even more critical. Recovery tends to be a greater challenge as you age, so taking advantage of this recovery support matters more for runners 50 and beyond.

This is not something you need to worry about after every run but only those runs that make demands on you and require more attention—think long runs, speed and hill work, and tempo runs (longer, harder efforts). Since recovery runs and easy aerobic runs should enhance your recovery, those do not call for this recovery protocol.

Massage

Massages generally feel great and reduce stress, which is always good for physical and mental recovery. But following a hard effort, your muscles can be a bit tender to the touch, so a massage after a hard race or workout likely won't feel the best. While studies are mixed concerning the benefits of massage, some suggest that joint ROM, flexibility, and muscle soreness improve after a massage. While there's no conclusive evidence that massage enhances performance, it may improve some of the more subjective issues after exercise (Davis et al. 2019). Also, having regular deep massage can make you aware of tight areas or muscle imbalances that you might otherwise not notice. These areas can lead to soreness and injury in the future if they are not addressed. Massage helps you check in with your body.

Anti-Inflammatory Medication

Many runners turn to nonsteroidal anti-inflammatory drugs (NSAIDs) to help relieve exercise-induced soreness and sometimes to alleviate pain caused by injuries. In both cases, this is a bad idea. Studies show that NSAIDs (ibuprofen, aspirin, Excedrin, etc.) actually inhibit recovery, removing the inflammatory process that is crucial to muscle repair (Mikkelsen et al. 2009). Remember that training causes an inflammatory response that prompts your body to repair. That's how you get stronger. Removing the inflammation removes the training stimulus—the signal telling your body to heal and get stronger based on the demands made on it.

Additionally, if you're taking an NSAID to dull the pain of an injury, you're likely to further hurt yourself because you don't feel that pain. Some take NSAIDs prophylactically, before races or hard workouts. This has been shown to be dangerous for your kidneys and can cause gastrointestinal distress. Tylenol (acetaminophen) is not an NSAID, so it can be used for pain management without some of the previously mentioned drawbacks—but you are more likely to do yourself more harm if you can't feel the pain response your body is trying to send.

Sleep

As I've mentioned many times up to this point, the most important part of recovery—and perhaps the key to a flourishing life—is adequate, quality sleep. How fast and how well you recover between hard workouts can make or break a training cycle. Recover well and quickly, and you may reap the benefits of hard runs. Recover poorly, and you will find yourself slipping into overtraining, exhaustion, chronic injuries, and frustrating fitness plateaus.

Sleep is the number one most important factor for recovery. Chronic low-level sleep deprivation leads to

> **Sleep is the number one most important factor for recovery.**

elevated levels of cortisol (a stress hormone) and a decrease in HGH, which may interfere with tissue repair and growth. Sleep is when HGH is most active. Glycogen synthesis also decreases because cortisol releases sugar into the system so that you can respond to stressful situations (fight or flight). All of this undermines adaptation. A study from 2018 found that HGH, which is necessary for muscle restoration and growth and bone building, is at its highest during non-rapid-eye-movement (non-REM) sleep (O'Donnell, Beaven, and Driller). While you may believe that sleep is just a time of rest, sleep is actually a very active time for your body, metabolically and hormonally. Each stage of sleep is crucial for recovery, repair, and restoration for your body and mind. Both sleep deprivation and interrupted sleep mean less time spent in non-REM sleep. Non-REM sleep is divided into three stages, and stage three is considered deep sleep, when most of the important work is done to repair and regenerate your body and brain (O'Donnell, Beaven, and Driller 2018).

And here's the kicker: While most adults require at least eight hours of sleep per day, athletes or those who are just very active during the day require more—upward of 8 to 10 hours of sleep per night. Research also indicates that not all sleep is equal. *When* you get sleep matters, and the more sleep you can get before midnight, the better. Sleeping from 9:00 p.m. to 6:00 a.m. allows for better, more restorative sleep than sleeping from midnight to 9:00 a.m. Additionally, many studies show that sleep medications undermine the quality of sleep.

As you get older, good sleep also becomes a bit more elusive. Older adults tend to take longer to fall asleep and tend to wake up earlier. This change can start in your 40s. Over time, sticking with old sleep patterns will interfere with both your physical and mental well-being (Chaput, Dutil, and Sampasa-Kanyinga 2018). As you age, stage-three non-REM (deep, slow-wave sleep) and REM sleep also tend to decrease (Li, Vitiello, and Gooneratne 2018). The problem here is not a couple nights of bad sleep. The problem is when you consistently get inadequate sleep. In a go-go-go culture, this is often the case for many of you. You make do with five to seven hours of sleep and soldier on. But this attitude undermines all your other efforts. Long-term inadequate sleep results in ongoing changes in hormone levels, particularly those related to stress and how you deal with stress, muscle recovery, and mood. Hence, there's a constant breakdown without the necessary rebuilding. Over time, this can lead to

> **Long-term inadequate sleep results in ongoing changes in hormone levels, particularly those related to stress and how you deal with stress, muscle recovery, and mood.**

injury and overtraining as you constantly make demands on your body but never allow for repair to take place.

Making sleep a priority, setting consistent sleep habits, removing all screens for 40 to 60 minutes before bed, and making your bedroom a bedroom only (not a place where you work or watch movies) all help in developing new and healthy sleep habits. There is one catch here, and it's that those who remain healthy (with few or no comorbidities) as they age appear to have fewer age-related sleep problems, suggesting that age alone is not the explanation for increased sleep difficulties. At the same time, quality sleep helps you stay healthy as you age. Age alone is not a predictor of poor sleep.

Recovery Tools

Since recovery is such an important part of any sport or exercise, it's also being heavily marketed as the population of athletes gets older. Companies see an opportunity to offer an ever-expanding array of gadgets to soothe your aching body, whether it's from doing too much exercise too soon or just daily wear and tear.

Companies are constantly rolling out new gadgets aimed at improving recovery time: recovery boots, rollers, massage balls, massage guns, TENS units, etc. Here's some information about each of these types of equipment so you can decide if they may help you.

Recovery Boots

Recovery boots, or external pneumatic compression boots, provide varied and graduated compression. Studies on recovery boots, like massage, are mixed—some show no performance or recovery benefit, and others show some improvement for delayed-onset muscle soreness (DOMS) (Haun et al. 2017). But they can feel good, so if that matters to you and it allows you to relax, and the cost is not an issue for you, then they certainly don't hurt and might help.

Massage Guns

Massage guns, or percussive massage devices, combine massage and vibration therapy and have been shown to help increase ROM and flexibility around joints (Konrad et al. 2020). A review of the literature on the effects of massage guns in physical therapy settings on flexibility and muscle strength suggests generally positive outcomes. The problem is that the research varies significantly in terms of the device used and the time applied. So, while percussive devices hold promise, there are still a lot of unknowns (Sams et al. 2023).

Cold-Water Immersion

In recent years, many runners have started using ice baths, or cold-water immersion (CWI), to help with recovery. While many studies show that CWI can reduce the symptoms of DOMS, lowering perceived soreness and stiffness, it has not been shown to actually reduce objective factors such as blood markers indicating inflammation. And recent studies suggest that CWI may interfere with the natural recovery and rebuilding process, which then undermines the idea that stress plus recovery equals increased strength. When your body repairs the damage done during a demanding workout or race, you end up stronger in the end. Artificially removing that damage removes the stimulus to grow stronger (like NSAIDS, discussed earlier). Recent studies show that ice baths inhibit recovery, decreasing both the body's anabolic responses to stress and protein muscle synthesis (Fuchs et al. 2020). This is exactly the opposite of what you want.

Rollers and Massagers

A meta-analysis of research on the effects of foam rollers and rolling massagers, such as trigger point balls, looks at both warm-up rolling before exercise and recovery rolling after exercise. What they found was that pre-exercise rolling increased sprint speed by a very small percentage. For an elite athlete, this might make the difference between winning and losing, but for recreational athletes, the improvement is not statistically significant. The mechanism involved in any enhancement is still speculative. Some suggestions are that rolling before a run breaks up trigger points; physically rolling on a foam roller requires muscular effort while supporting your body, thus warming up the muscles and your core temperature (similar to planking); and there may even be a psychological (placebo) effect because the athlete believes it helps. But what is observed is a statistically significant increase in short-term flexibility and a reduction in pain sensations. For older runners, this is something to pay attention to. Postrun rolling has been shown to enhance recovery. For pre-exercise rolling, both foam rollers and rolling massagers have similar results, but for postrun rolling, foam rollers appear to offer greater benefits. However, more research needs to be done (Wiewelhove et al. 2019).

Compression Clothing

Makers of compression clothing make claims about recovery and minimizing muscle damage during exercise by reducing muscle vibration. Current research shows this claim to be nothing more than pseudoscience. Remember that exercise is supposed to damage muscle a little bit. That's what the body repairs to become stronger. Does compression clothing enhance recovery? That is still being studied, and some research shows some beneficial effects postexercise (Beliard et al. 2015). However, most commercial compression clothing marketed to athletes varies greatly in terms of how much pressure is applied. At this time, the best that can be said is that compression gear may help with recovery. Like recovery boots, compression clothing can *feel* good, so that's a benefit if that applies to you.

Recovery tools certainly have a place in enhancing recovery time and preventing injury. These tools—along with dynamic stretching, drills, and static stretching—can be part of your toolbox for healthy running. Used correctly, they can make you more mindful of self-care and can also alert you to sore areas that might otherwise go unnoticed and be allowed to fester into a problem. However, sometimes devices are marketed as panaceas, promising to remedy every ache and pain while improving health and performance. As always, buyer beware of these grandiose claims. If it sounds too good to be true, it probably is.

As I mentioned at the start of this chapter, there's the day-to-day, month-to-month, and year-to-year recovery to include in your annual plan, and then there's recovery that follows a period of training for a specific goal before moving on to a new goal.

Recovery During a Transition Period

Transition periods are times at the end of or between training cycles or during what is sometimes called offseason. Basically, it's a little lull in your training or racing. It can be scheduled annually, or it can be based on how you plan your training to reach your goals (these need not be race goals). For example, as a coach, I often schedule transition periods for my clients after big goal races and before another training cycle begins. Transitions entail recovery and then rebuilding, but the recovery comes first. Let's say you just ran your goal race for the fall. You've been training hard for several months, maybe throwing in some tune-up races, and now you aren't sure what to do with yourself. Here's a look at how some runners tend to approach this postseason recovery (this is what I hear from so many runners):

Coming Off a Good Race or Season

When runners are coming off a good race or season, they often think things like

I can't stop now!

I'm in great shape!

I need to build on this!

I can't lose what's taken so long to achieve!

I want more! I must do more!

And so, the usual approach looks something like this: For a couple days, you rest. Perhaps you go for a walk or a swim or dust off the bike for a ride. But after a couple days, you're itching to run. You're losing fitness. You feel it oozing from your pores. You see your legs getting soft. Sure, you had a good race. But that postrace glow fades fast. Two days ago, you were ecstatic. Life was great. The world was a bright and happy place. Today, you woke up unable to drag your sorry butt out from under the covers. You are depressed. You are floating in a sea of ambiguity. What now? Postmarathon blues have hit with a vengeance.

Coming Off a Disappointing Race or Season

When runners are coming off a disappointing race or season, they often think things like

I didn't work very hard.

I don't deserve to rest.

I wasted all that training. I need to do something with it.

Since that didn't work, I just need to work harder.

And so, the usual approach looks something like this: For a couple days, you fester and try to find some silver lining—some lesson learned or some positive something. You may feel tired, but that's just weakness manifested; it's not real, deserved fatigue. Soon, you are back out there, having decided on a new goal or trying to beat your weary body into submission. Whatever you did didn't work. The only answer is to hit it harder.

These approaches generally work for about 7 to 14 days before you start declining (results may vary). At some point, usually during week two or three, you feel exactly zero motivation to ever run again. Every run feels like a herculean effort—physically, psychologically, and emotionally. Then you beat yourself up for not wanting it more. Thus ensues a vicious circle that lasts a week, a month, a year, or more.

I encourage runners of all ages, but especially those over 50, to take a serious physical and mental break after finishing a training cycle—or just after months of steady running. If you're running marathons or ultras, that can mean a month or more of much lower volume and lower-intensity running. A forced rest due to injury does not count for this intentional downtime. This should be something that you schedule into your year every year.

While different times of year will work better for different people, find that time of year where you just want to chill a bit. Pick four weeks, and make that your recovery cycle. As an example: I like to take time off during November and December. Where I live, this is the darkest time of the year, and it's also a busy time with holidays and family and work responsibilities. Because I schedule this time into my plan, I actually look forward to it. Many of my coached runners also like taking this as a little downtime; fall races are generally completed, and they can use this time to recharge before the new year. Some of my runners prefer taking time off during the summer months due to vacations or hot weather. Whatever time works for your life schedule will work best for this. It's important to understand that this will keep you healthier and more motivated in the long run.

This is the perfect time to mix in some cross-training or focus on developing a new skill. Keep in mind that recovery does not just mean rest—as in, doing nothing. Some forms of active recovery, such as swimming, have been shown to actually improve recovery times (Lum, Landers, and Peeling 2010). Biking, hiking, walking, stand-up paddleboarding, or kayaking can be some fun new activities to add that allow your body to recover from running stresses while still maintaining a base level of fitness.

Rest and recovery must be part of your weekly, monthly, and yearly plan. Recovery is not the absence of training but part of training. This is when the adaptations happen—when your body is able to respond to the work you've done to grow stronger. Adding in some restorative support such as massage, warm baths, light rolling, meditation, good sleep and nutrition, or anything that you find reduces stress will maximize your body's ability to adapt quickly. Take your recovery as seriously as you take the work. Recovery plays a crucial role in optimizing performance, preventing injuries and burnout, and promoting overall health and well-being.

PART III

PROGRAMMING

Chapter 8

Creating Your Training Plan

Running is easy—or so it seems. The challenge for most is figuring out the how with all this. Regardless of your goals, if you want to run, for whatever reason speaks to you, how do you do it? How do you reach your goals? How do you start? How do you improve? How do you continue, over days and weeks and years and decades? What should you do today, tomorrow, next month, and next year to achieve the things you want to achieve?

Some like to say, "Just run." But often, just running leads to injury, a feeling that you aren't progressing, and confusion about what to do next. Understanding how to plan things, balance stresses, and decide what to do now and in the coming months is not as simple as just running. Having some idea of how best to plan and organize your training in a periodized way will keep you healthy and moving in the direction you desire.

No matter where you begin, when you set off on a new challenge, you need to take the long view. It doesn't matter whether you're aiming to complete your first 5K or your 50th marathon, smart training applies to you. You must start from where you are now and aim at where you might want to be in the future.

Don'ts When Creating Your Training Plan

There are several common mistakes I see runners making time and again—both newer and more experienced runners. These mistakes happen when you don't understand the purpose of a particular run or the organization of different sorts of runs over time. Many don't know there are different kinds of runs based on pace or effort, distance, terrain, weather, and other factors. Understanding what you're trying to accomplish and how you will be able to accomplish it will help you avoid these mistakes.

Doing Too Much Too Soon

Imagine you start walking a mile every day. Things feel good, so the second week, you do two miles of walk-run intervals each day. By week three, feeling excited about your progress, you move to three miles of walk-run intervals and add in three 30-minute sessions of resistance training at the gym. On Monday morning, you try to get out of bed only to find that every muscle in your body aches. You notice sharp pains in your shins that leave you hobbling through your day. You take the day off to rest, but the next day, the pain still leaves you cringing with every step. This continues for the next week. You try again the next week, only to discover half a mile in that you cannot go on. You slowly walk home, feeling defeated and frustrated. It takes several weeks for this to finally settle down. Now you find yourself back at your starting place.

Progressive overload entails adding small increments of physical demands over time, allowing time for adaptation, adding a bit more demand, allowing adaptation, and repeating the cycle. What those increments of demand are will depend on your goals, your health, your time, your desire, and your exercise history. The problem with doing too much too fast is that you add stress faster than your body can recover and adapt, so you end up tearing yourself down over time instead of building yourself up. Progressive overload demands that you add enough stress but not too much stress. That is the difficult part. Do too little, and progress is painfully slow. Do too much, and you break down. What you need to find is just the right balance. The safest way to do this is to incorporate recovery days and recovery weeks. Combining harder days and easier days is also a way to avoid injury.

Let's revisit the above scenario: In week one, you walk a mile each on Monday, Wednesday, and Saturday. You walk half a mile on both Tuesday and Sunday, and you take a complete rest day on Friday. In week two, you walk a mile and a half on your longer days but keep the recovery days and rest day unchanged. In week three, you keep all the distances the same but add in some running intervals on your longer days. Notice that there are ebbs and flows here—hard days, easy days, days that you build upon, and days that you hold steady. Importantly, any change is focused on only one element. In the example, everything is held steady except the harder day—and as speed is added (the running intervals), the distance is held steady. If you add strength training along the way, you would add that to the harder days while holding the runs and walks steady, and you would add that progressively as well. While this may sound like a tedious process, it will allow you to avoid the injury-recovery-restart cycle that undermines the number one principle of improvement—consistency.

Expecting Too Much Too Soon

Say you start off walking a mile every other day. The next week, you add an extra day, but the following morning, you wake up feeling sore and fatigued. You wonder why you aren't getting anywhere with your new exercise regimen. Instead of listening to your body and backing off just a bit to allow yourself a little extra rest, you quit, feeling discouraged and weak.

In running, improvement takes time and patience. You are building not just your muscles, tendons, and ligaments but also your cardiorespiratory, nervous, digestive, and metabolic systems. As an example, muscles grow stronger relatively quickly. But tendons and ligaments develop strength more slowly. Unrealistic expectations set you up for frustration and disappointment. Realistic expectations set the stage for success. Setting reasonable fitness goals, with benchmark goals along the way, allows you to measure and celebrate your progress.

Doing the Same Thing

Suppose you've been running for a couple months. Right now, you are running three miles, five days a week. You feel like you're getting nowhere as your paces stay the same day after day, and you can't seem to run any farther than three miles. How do you break out of this stagnation?

Doing the same thing every day leads to stagnation because you're training the same things all the time. What you're doing every day will elicit the same training response every time, and your body has already adapted to the stress you're placing on it. The result is that you are in a holding pattern. You're maintaining what you've built thus far, but you aren't adding more, and so you will stay where you are now.

The solution to this problem is to vary the stresses: harder days and easier days, longer days and shorter days, faster days and slower days, adding either volume or speed incrementally. This keeps things fresh, adds beneficial stresses, and leads to improvement in fitness.

Making Every Day a Time Trial

This is a variation of the previous scenario, where you run the same route every day, but your goal every single day is to run that route faster than the day before. You believe that running as fast as you can every day is the only way to get faster. This results in slower times instead of faster times—and with that, frustration.

Racing every run means shortchanging your aerobic development. Running anything longer than 300 meters is primarily aerobic, and your aerobic engine is best developed by running comfortable paces. Trying to race every run has you working hard every run—which may sound good, but it means you're only developing a narrow part of your running physiology. On top of that, think about what you're asking your body to do: run just a little faster every day. Every day is a test of fitness. The days you manage to run faster, you win. The days you do not run faster, you fail. That's all the feedback you see or care about.

Goals need to be measurable and reasonable. Having indeterminate goals or measurements never lets you get anywhere. With this approach, there is no plan except for today's goal—which is to run faster than yesterday—and each day, the goal is the same.

The solution is to set goalposts along the way, perhaps a series of time trials spaced out every month or two, while using well-rounded training stimuli that will get you to your tests ready to give it your best.

Dos When Creating Your Training Plan

When putting together a training plan, there are some important concepts to keep in mind to achieve progressive overload (how you get stronger and faster) and avoid injury and overtraining. The first is balancing stress and rest, which I've emphasized throughout this book. Training well lets you gradually increase stress (training load) and allow for adaptation. Rest and recovery along with progressive overload maximizes the training stimulus and the adaptation. Practices that help you tolerate and optimize stress and recovery reap the greatest benefits in terms of improving your fitness for running and continuing to be active and healthy as you get older.

Including a Proper Warm-Up

An easy 10 to 15 minutes of dynamic drills followed by some easy jogging helps prepare both your mind and your body for activity. This is true not only for races but for everyday training as well. While warm-ups may not be as important for recovery runs since those are run at a very easy rate of perceived exertion, there's no harm in doing some drills even before setting out on an easy run. A warm-up does the following:

- *Increases blood flow:* A warm-up gradually increases your heart rate and your body temperature, which in turn increases blood flow to your muscles. This boosts the delivery of oxygen and nutrients to your muscles.
- *Improves muscle elasticity:* Warm muscles, tendons, and ligaments are all more elastic and pliable, reducing the risk of injury during exercise. Increased blood flow and temperature allow muscles to contract with greater force and speed.
- *Enhances joint flexibility and mobility:* Warming up increases synovial fluid, which lubricates the joints.
- *Prepares cardiorespiratory system:* As your heart rate and respiratory rate gradually rise, this prepares your cardiorespiratory system for the demands of running.
- *Activates nervous system:* A warm-up helps activate the nervous system, which improves coordination, reaction time, and mental awareness and gets you into a rhythm.

Many wonder why static stretching is discouraged while dynamic stretching and drills are encouraged before exercise. Static stretching (holding a stretched position for a period of time) prior to running actually impairs performance due to a reduction in both muscle strength and power (Chaabene et al. 2019). While static stretching, done correctly, may increase ROM, it also decreases musculotendinous stiffness. This may sound good—after all, you don't want to be overly tight—but prior to a workout or race, you don't want your muscles overly stretched. Running requires muscular contraction, so muscle turgidity is actually a good thing going into a run. Dynamic stretches and warm-up drills before a run help prepare your muscles for the work ahead. These drills involve moving joints through their full ROM, adding in some gait cues, and firing up the muscles, tendons, and ligaments.

Here is an example of a dynamic warm-up composed of simple and common exercises that I often use with my athletes:

1. Walking deadlifts (10 to 20 reps)
2. Knee hugs (10 to 20 reps)
3. Donkey kicks (10 reps with each leg)
4. Mountain climbers (10 to 20 reps with leg in and leg out)
5. Iron cross (20 reps)
6. Forward lunge (10 reps)
7. Twisting lunge (10 reps)
8. Side lunge (10 reps)
9. Diagonal lunge (10 reps)
10. Backward lunge (10 reps)
11. Front leg swing (10 reps with each leg)
12. Side leg swing (10 reps with each leg)

Being Consistent yet Flexible

Any plan that works for you will allow some degree of flexibility. With the plans presented in the next two chapters, you have several recovery or rest days to either take extra rest when needed or to shift things around based on other life demands. The schedules can be shifted based on what days work better for you. For example, if you would rather have Sundays off, shift everything forward a day. Whatever day you wish to have as a rest day, you can adjust the plan with that in mind.

You may also prefer to make one of the recovery run days a cross-training day. If you choose to do that, base your cross-training duration on your normal run duration for that day—so if your run takes 40 minutes, cross-train for 40 minutes. Remember, recovery days are for *recovery*. These are not days to add a different hard workout such as heavy lifting, CrossFit, or HIIT.

Finally, if you miss a run, do not try to make up for lost time. Simply continue with the plan. If you need to miss several days for injury or illness, pull back a bit and gradually get yourself back to where you were. How quickly that should be depends on how long you've had to rest. A few days will have little impact, but a week or more will require adjustments. So, if you miss a week or two of training, it's best to go back a week or even two in your training plan.

Learning How to Fuel Your Run

Part of training is learning how to fuel. You should be training with the fuel you plan to use during the race you're training for. If you prefer using the fuel offered on the course, practice using it to see if it agrees with you. Different fuel works for different people, in terms of both taste preference and what agrees with your stomach—but once you find something you like, here are some general guidelines to keep in mind:

- Aim for 150 to 300 calories an hour. Through your training, you will discover what works best for you. Pay particular attention to what's working for faster runs. But understand that you are also training your gut to tolerate the fuel. As you do that, what you can tolerate may increase.
- For marathons and shorter runs, liquids, gels, and chews generally work best because you will likely be running at a pace that makes digesting real food more difficult. It is very important to note that you must take gels with water. Do not take gels alone, and do not take them with liquid calories. Your gut can only process so many carbs at one time, so if you consume too many at once, the carbs are just going to sit there and wreak havoc on your gastrointestinal system.
- For any run over an hour, practice fueling. Fine-tune your fueling during training, not during the race.

Including Time for Rest and Recovery

Make rest and recovery a key part of your training plan. Again, remember that recovery is training, not the absence of it (see chapter 7). It's a necessary part of a good training plan. This means it must be part of your weekly, monthly, and annual plans. Recovery can be an easy run or some other easy activity. It does not need to be complete rest, but it needs to be very easy. In most cases, if you do a recovery activity, you should feel better at the end of it than you did at the beginning. Think about how it feels when you stand up after sitting for a long time and then go for a walk—after a few minutes of walking, you feel so much better. That's what you're after.

Incorporating Gradual Progressive Overload

When increasing training stress, it's important to keep track of both volume (miles over time, most easily measured over a week) and intensity, including speed work (strides, intervals, repeats, tempo runs) and hill work (hill repeats, increased elevation runs, downhill running). It is best to add either volume or intensity but not both at the same time. Let's say you're at a point where you want to add some speed after building your volume. Keep the volume (weekly mileage) steady and add some intensity one day a week to start. This could be as simple as adding some fast one-minute strides to an aerobic run or throwing in some fartleks ("speed play" of varying speeds and distances, but usually short bursts of speed). Importantly, you do not want to increase your total volume and speed dramatically.

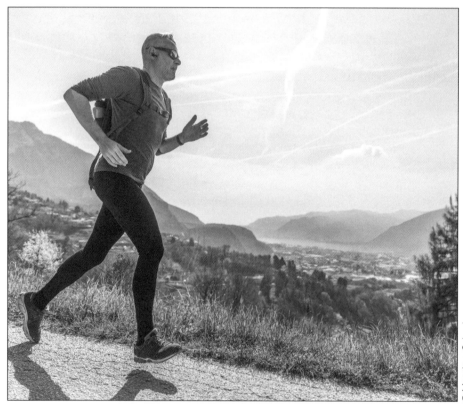

How to Choose a Training Plan That Is Right for You

So far, you've learned about how training works in general and the basic setup for training plans. Many runners choose training plans spanning a set number of weeks working toward a specific goal. These set plans have their advantages:

- They allow you to see what is expected of you from the start of the plan to the conclusion.
- They are cost-effective; many are either free or low-cost.
- They provide basic guidance on how to organize a training cycle.

However, set plans can also have some disadvantages:

- They don't change based on how you are responding to the training.
- They can be difficult to adjust around other life demands—work, family, vacation, illness, or injury.

When choosing a set training plan, try to pick one you believe will work with your life rather than trying to work your life around the training plan. Yes, if this is important to you, you do need to make some choices and a commitment to doing the work. Most of you have busy lives with work, family, and other demands. Based on my decades of experience working with runners, I know there is no such thing as finding time. You have to *make* time if it matters; you can always make time for the things that matter. For example, if you have a very demanding schedule, hiring a coach may be the best choice for you. A coach can help you adjust your running schedule to maximize training and results while balancing your other commitments.

There are some important aspects of training to keep in mind when using a set training plan. Do not try to make up for a missed run. If you miss a run, trying to add to your next run may not be a good idea. If you miss a recovery run, it's usually best to just let that go and move on. If you miss a longer run, perhaps a run that has been building for several weeks, it's better to take a conservative approach. Do not add mileage or intensity too quickly. Let go of the missed run and move on. If you miss training for illness, vacation, family, or work demands and this extends for a week or more, do not just jump back into the plan where you should be for that week. Go back to where you left off—and possibly farther. This really depends on how much you've missed. But always keep in mind that it is better to do too little in this case than to do too much. Remember that consistency is the key to ongoing improvement. Injuries interrupt this consistency more than any other factor.

I want to mention two important points about training in general: (1) Longer does not equal better (more on that later), so a half-marathon is not better than a 5K, and (2) while gradually increasing race distance is not necessary, if you have longer goals, you will learn a lot as you progress on your running journey.

Let's say you've started walking and maybe adding in some short jogs. You've been doing this consistently for several weeks or maybe several months. The idea of a 5K pops into your head, and it sounds kind of intriguing. Now, how do you get there? When training for your first 5K, you will learn how your body responds to increases in training demands. You will also build a deeper foundation of aerobic fitness as you train. You can then build on what you've learned and on your developing fitness. There are many options from here, including setting time goals for your next 5K or moving up from a 5K to a 10K. This process of building speed and distance can continue depending on your goals.

Remember that training plans are like road maps: They can guide you to where you want to be. Taking shortcuts, skipping ahead, or going off the plan can lead you down a different path. Take it day by day and week by week.

Being consistent, having patience, and listening to your body will get you to your goals, but always remember that the process matters. Enjoy the process. Take note of your progress along the way. Notice that each day offers an opportunity to learn, achieve, improve, and discover new aspects of yourself and the world around you. In the process, you will discover more opportunities to follow, new goals to pursue, and different paths to explore.

Chapter 9

5K, 10K, and Half-Marathon Training Plans

The training plans provided here can serve many purposes. They can build your running base with fun race goals along the way. The beginner plans can be used like a couch-to-5K plan or for improvement on past race results. These plans can also be incorporated into an annual plan when you want to switch your training up, perhaps focusing on 5Ks or 10Ks between marathon training cycles. What's great about middle-distance races is that you can run quite a few of them over the course of a year. Recovery time for these races is considerably shorter than for marathons, so shorter races allow you to work on speed and hone your race logistics. Becoming comfortable in a race situation will help you whether your goals are 5Ks or 100-milers.

For those who tend to gravitate toward longer races, adding a couple yearly cycles of shorter, faster racing can really push you out of your comfort zone while also introducing fun, social racing. For those who are newer to running, 5Ks, 10Ks and even half-marathons present ambitious goals, direction for your training and fitness building, and fun social events. What's great about racing is that it does not matter how fast or slow you go; you will find a place in the race and others doing the same to share the experience with.

5K, 10K, and Half-Marathon Training: General Terms and Recommendations

Before we get into the plans, there are some general recommendations and nomenclature you need to know that are specific to the 5K, 10K, and half-marathon training plans:

- Each day should begin with an easy dynamic warm-up (see exercises in chapter 8) followed by 10 minutes of easy running—no static stretching before running! For race-day warm-ups, the shorter the race, the longer the warm-up. For less experienced runners, a warm-up of one to two miles for a 5K and one mile for a 10K is plenty. I don't recommend more than a five-minute warm-up for a half-marathon; use the first two to three miles of the race to gradually increase your pace.

- Strides are fast, controlled accelerations. These are short and based on effort. Add in 20 seconds of jogging or walking between each acceleration. This is the only speed work included in the beginner plan.

- On the days you only walk, these are steady walks, but you don't need to worry about how fast they are. They should be at a pressing effort—not just a casual stroll.

- While there are no specific strength workouts prescribed in these plans, there are two principles to keep in mind: (1) Lift heavy—a weight you cannot lift for more than 8 to 12 repetitions or repeats. For a set, do 2 or 3 × 8 to 12 repetitions of each exercise. (2) Hit the seven basic movement patterns: pull, press or push, carry, lunge, squat, rotation, and hinge.

- On the days you do a run and strength work, ideally you should do your run first—you are training for running, after all!—and then strength work after. It's best to do it several hours after your run, but if time doesn't permit this, do it when you can.
- On the days you cross-train, choose your preferred cross-training for the time noted. Cross-training options include biking, swimming, using an elliptical, rowing, in-line skating, walking, and hiking, all at an aerobic effort—conversational and comfortable, but your body is still working.
- General aerobic runs, the bulk of your training, should feel comfortable. You should be able to carry on a conversation while running and not hear yourself breathing.
- Easy, or recovery, runs should be at a leisurely pace. You really can't run these too slow. Feel free to sing a song or walk if you feel like taking in a beautiful sunrise or sunset. You should feel better after the run than you did before.
- Hard-effort runs should feel like you're pushing beyond a comfortable pace. You will not be able to talk easily, and you will hear yourself breathing.
- Cutdown runs are a specific type of tempo run—a pace you can maintain for 60 minutes—that build faster as the run progresses. Begin at your aerobic pace, and run each mile 10 to 20 seconds faster than the previous mile. The aim is to work down to your goal race pace, or even a bit faster, by the final mile.
- Progression runs are done at a general aerobic pace for the first half or so and then at a slightly faster pace for the rest.
- Race-pace runs include a set number of miles at your goal race pace within a general aerobic run.
- Hill repeats are short (100 to 300 meters max) and are run on a moderately steep hill at a fast, pressing pace.
- Hill circuits are 200 to 800 meters long on a moderate hill. The number of repeats depends on the estimated length of the hill you use. This is how you perform a circuit:
  - Run strong up the hill—not a sprint, just a slightly pressing effort.
  - Jog for two to four minutes at the top.
  - Run down the hill quick and light.
  - Jog for three to four minutes at the bottom.
  - Run for 5 to 10 minutes at your general aerobic pace or until you reach the designated distance noted for the run.
- Hilly fartleks are performed by choosing a moderately hilly route and pushing some of the uphills faster as you feel like it. Do not sprint the hills—just run at a pushing pace.

(continued)

**5K, 10K, and Half-Marathon Training:
General Terms and Recommendations** *(continued)*

- Intervals are run at a hard pace but not an all-out effort—you should be able to get a word or two out (80 percent effort). You won't be fully recovered between faster segments.
- Repeats are run at a very hard effort, and you won't be able to talk (90 to 100 percent effort). The aim is complete recovery between harder bouts of running, but the faster segments are all-out efforts.
- Sprint-floats are a type of surge-and-glide run. These are best done on a 400-meter track; you sprint, or surge, on the 100-meter straightaway and float, or glide, around the turns. Run continuously and aim for an effort where you can maintain a consistent pace on the sprint segments for the entire workout without stopping to rest. Part of the challenge is to find a pace that is fast but not too fast. If your pace drops or your form begins breaking down, then this workout is done. If you don't have access to a track or it's difficult to get to, these can be done with a bit less precision on a flat road.
- With any speed work, you should end the workout when your form breaks down in any way or when your split time drops significantly.
- Taper runs use either a general aerobic or easy aerobic pace (noted in the plan). Remember, volume decreases but intensity remains steady during a taper.
- Shakeout runs are performed the day before a race to get the blood moving and to help with prerace nervous energy. They should be run at a very comfortable pace and end with some short, fast strides.
- Regardless of the research, many runners prefer a cooldown of easier running to slowly back off after a hard effort, allowing their heart rate to lower and their breathing to settle. There seems to be at least a mental, if not a physiological, reason for a cooldown. Based on empirical observations, I often include an easier run to wrap up the workout.

Beginner 5K and 10K Training Plans

The focus of the beginner 5K and 10K training plans is to increase your aerobic engine, which requires comfortable mileage. As discussed in chapter 5, this is the foundation for all running. These plans include a mix of running and walking if you so desire. Unless otherwise noted, they are done at a conversational pace, meaning you can easily carry on a conversation while running or walking. Whether your aim is to move toward all running or a combination of running and walking is a personal choice. If, however, you are adding in walk intervals because you cannot continue running, you will need to slow down your run segments and allow time to build your aerobic fitness.

The beginner 5K plan is for someone who is just starting to run, returning to running after a long break, or wants to try out a race for the first time (figure 9.1). There's no minimum weekly mileage to start the beginner 5K plan. The beginner 10K training plan (figure 9.2) builds on the 5K plan or assumes you have been running or walking consistently for three months or more, averaging a minimum of 10 miles a week.

Figure 9.1 Beginner 5K Training Plan

Week	Mon	Tues	Wed	Thurs	Fri	Sat	Sun	Total
1	Rest	20 min, run or walk	Strength training	20 min, run or walk	Rest	30 min, run or walk	20 min, walk	90 min
2	Rest	30 min, run or walk	Strength training	30 min, run or walk	Rest	40 min, run or walk	30 min, walk	130 min
3	Rest	40 min, run or walk	Rest	40 min, run or walk	Rest	50 min, run or walk Strength training	30 min, walk	160 min
4 (recovery)	Rest	30 min, run or walk	Strength training	30 min, run or walk	Rest	40 min, run or walk	30 min, walk	130 min
5	Rest	2 miles, run or walk Strength training	1 mile, run or walk	2 miles, run or walk	Rest	3 miles, run or walk Strength training	30 min, cross-train	8 miles + 30 min
6	Rest	2 miles, run or walk Strength training	1 mile, run or walk	2 miles, run or walk	Rest	3.5 miles, run or walk Strength training	40 min, cross-train	8.5 miles + 40 min
7 (recovery)	Rest	1.75 miles, run or walk Strength training	1 mile, run or walk	1.75 miles, run or walk	Rest	2.5 miles, run or walk Strength training	40 min, cross-train	7 miles + 40 min
8	Rest	2 miles, run or walk Strength training	1.5 miles, run or walk	2 miles, run or walk	Rest	3.5 miles, run or walk Strength training	50 min, cross-train	9 miles + 50 min
9	Rest	2 miles, run or walk Strength training	1.5 miles, run or walk	2 miles, run or walk	Rest	2.5 miles, run or walk Strength training	20 min, cross-train	8 miles + 20 min
10 (taper)	Rest	1.5 miles, run or walk	Rest	1.5 miles, run or walk	Rest	1 mile, easy shakeout	Race day!	4 miles + race

Figure 9.2 Beginner 10K Training Plan

Week	Mon	Tues	Wed	Thurs	Fri	Sat	Sun	Total
1	Rest	3 miles, run or walk Strength training	2 miles, run or walk	3 miles, run or walk	Rest	3 miles, run or walk Strength training	30 min, walk	11 miles + 30 min
2	Rest	3.5 miles, run or walk Strength training	2 miles, run or walk	3.5 miles, run or walk	Rest	4 miles, run or walk Strength training	30 min, walk	13 miles + 30 min
3	Rest	3.5 miles, run or walk Strength training	2 miles, run or walk	4 miles, run or walk	Rest	5 miles, run or walk Strength training	30 min, walk	14.5 miles + 30 min
4 (recovery)	Rest	2 miles, run or walk	30 min, walk	2 miles, run or walk	Rest	3 miles, run or walk	30 min, walk	7 miles + 1 hr
5	Rest	4 miles, run or walk 3 × 20 sec strides to finish Strength training	2 miles, run or walk	4 miles, run or walk 3 × 20 sec strides to finish Strength training	Rest	5 miles, run or walk Strength training	30 min, cross-train	15 miles + 30 min
6	Rest	4 miles, run or walk 3 × 20 sec strides to finish Strength training	2 miles, run or walk	4 miles, run or walk 3 × 20 sec strides to finish Strength training	Rest	5.5 miles, run or walk Strength training	40 min, cross-train	15.5 miles + 40 min
7 (recovery)	Rest	3 miles, run or walk Strength training	2 miles, run or walk	3 miles, run	Rest	4 miles, run Strength training	50 min, cross-train	12 miles + 50 min
8	Rest	4.5 miles, run 3 × 20 sec strides to finish Strength training	2 miles, run or walk	4.5 miles, run 3 × 20 sec strides to finish	Rest	6.5 miles, run Strength training	50 min, cross-train	17.5 miles + 50 min
9	Rest	4 miles, run 3 × 20 sec strides to finish Strength training	2 miles, run or walk	4 miles, run 3 × 20 sec strides to finish	Rest	5 miles, run	20 min, cross-train	15 miles + 20 min
10 (taper)	Rest	3 miles, run or walk	Rest	2.5 miles, run or walk	Rest	2 miles, run or walk shakeout	Race day!	7.5 miles + race

For the week after your 5K, allow at least two days for easy active recovery, such as 20 minutes of swimming, biking, or walking. Then begin working runs and walks back into your schedule gradually. Return to a base level consistent with week five in the training plan. Spend some time thinking about what your next goal might be—perhaps a faster 5K or even a 10K.

Intermediate 5K and 10K Training Plans

The intermediate 5K and 10K plans (figure 9.3) are for runners who have run these distances before (either in races or on your own) and are looking to run the distances faster or stronger, cut out walk breaks, or run a harder course. These plans assume that, from the start, you are able to finish a three- to four-mile run for the 5K plan and a six- to seven-mile run for the 10K plan. You should also be averaging at least 8 to 10 miles a week for the 5K plan and 12 to 15 miles a week for the 10K plan.

For the 5K plan, aim for the low end of the mileage range given; for the 10K plan, aim for the high end of the mileage range given. This means that if a run specifies 8 to 13 miles, the 5K runner will run 8 to 10 miles, and the 10K runner will run 11 to 13 miles. For the 10K plan, you have one 5K race three weeks out from your goal race. This should be run at a hard effort, but start out comfortably and press the pace faster with each mile—the last 800 meters or half mile should be run at 90 percent effort.

Figure 9.3 Intermediate 5K and 10K Training Plan

Week	Mon	Tues	Wed	Thurs	Fri	Sat	Sun	Total
1	Rest	2-3 miles, general aerobic run Strength training	1-2 miles, recovery run	2-3 miles, general aerobic run	Rest	3-5 miles, general aerobic run Strength training	30 min, cross-train	8-13 miles + 30 min
2	Rest	2.5-4 miles, general aerobic run Strength training	2 miles, recovery run	2.5-4 miles, general aerobic run	Rest	4-6 miles, general aerobic run Strength training	30 min, cross-train	11-16 miles + 30 min
3	Rest	3-5 miles, hill circuits Strength training	2 miles, easy run or walk	3-5 miles, general aerobic run	Rest	5-7 miles, general aerobic run Strength training	40 min, cross-train	13-19 miles + 40 min

(continued)

Figure 9.3 Intermediate 5K and 10K Training Plan *(continued)*

Week	Mon	Tues	Wed	Thurs	Fri	Sat	Sun	Total
4 (recovery)	Rest	1.5-3 miles, general aerobic run	1-2 miles, recovery run	1.5-3 miles, general aerobic run Strength training	Rest	2-4 miles, general aerobic run	30 min, cross-train	6-12 miles + 30 min
5	Rest	3.5-5 miles, hill circuits Strength training	2 miles, run or walk	3.5-5 miles, progression run Strength training	Rest	6-8 miles, general aerobic run Strength training	40 min, cross-train	15-20 miles + 40 min
6	Rest	4-6 miles, hill repeats: 5-10 × 100-300 m with walk to the start for recovery Strength training	2 miles, run or walk	4-6 miles, progression run 3 × 20 sec strides to finish Strength training	Rest	7-10 miles, general aerobic run Strength training	40 min, cross-train	17-24 miles + 40 min
7 (recovery)	Rest	3-4 miles, general aerobic run Strength training	2 miles, recovery run	3-4 miles, general aerobic run	Rest	5-7 miles, general aerobic run Strength training	30 min, cross-train	13-17 miles + 30 min
8	Rest	4.5-7 miles, speed run: 10-min easy warm-up with 3 × 20 sec strides to finish 5 × 200-m hard-effort run with 200-m recovery jog/walk 10-15 min aerobic run to finish Strength training	2 miles, run or walk	5-7 miles, cutdown run: 1 mile, easy run 3-5 miles, cutdown 1 mile, cooldown Strength training	Rest	5K plan: 8 miles, progression run 10K plan: 5K race: 1 mile, warm-up 5K, race pace 1 mile, cooldown 3 × 20 sec strides to finish Strength training	50 min, cross-train	19.5-27 miles + 50 min

Week	Mon	Tues	Wed	Thurs	Fri	Sat	Sun	Total
				DAY				
9	Rest	5-6 miles, speed run: 10-min easy warm-up with 3 × 20 sec strides to finish 6-7 × 200-m hard-effort run with 200-m recovery jog 10-15 min aerobic run to finish Strength training	1.5-2 miles, run or walk	5-7 miles, cutdown run: 1 mile, easy run 3-5 miles, cutdown 1 mile, cooldown	Rest	5-7 miles, general aerobic run 3 × 20 sec strides to finish	50 min, cross-train	16.5-22 miles + 50 min
10 (taper)	Rest	1.5-4 miles, general aerobic run and speed work: 6 × 100-m fast-effort run (80%) with 100-m easy recovery jog	30 min, easy cross-train	1.5-3 miles, general aerobic run	Rest	1-3 miles, shakeout run	Race day!	4-10 miles + 30 min + race

Advanced 5K and 10K Training Plans

The advanced plans (figures 9.4 and 9.5) are for runners who have run these distances before (either in races or on your own) and are looking to run the distances faster or stronger, cut out walk breaks, or run a harder course. Remember, these are *your* goals.

Figure 9.4 Advanced 5K Training Plan

Week	Mon	Tues	Wed	Thurs	Fri	Sat	Sun	Total
				DAY				
1	3 miles, recovery run	4 miles, hill circuits Strength training	3 miles, recovery run	4 miles, general aerobic run	Rest	4 miles, progression run	5 miles, general aerobic run Strength training	23 miles

(continued)

Figure 9.4 Advanced 5K Training Plan *(continued)*

Week	Mon	Tues	Wed	Thurs	Fri	Sat	Sun	Total
2	3 miles, recovery run	4 miles, hill circuits Strength training	3 miles, recovery run	4 miles, general aerobic run Strength training	Rest	5 miles, cutdown run: 1 mile, easy 3 miles, cutdown 1 mile, cooldown	6 miles, general aerobic run Strength training	25 miles
3	3 miles, recovery run	5 miles, hill repeats: 5-10 × 100-300 m with walk to the start for recovery Strength training	3 miles, recovery run	5 miles, general aerobic run Strength training	Rest	5 miles, cutdown run: 1 mile, easy 3 miles, cutdown 1 mile, cooldown	7 miles, general aerobic run Strength training	28 miles
4 (recovery)	3 miles, recovery run	4 miles, speed work: 1 mile, easy 2 miles, sprint-floats for 10 × 100 m 1 mile, general aerobic run to finish	3 miles, recovery run	3 miles, general aerobic run with 3 × 20 sec strides to finish Strength training	Rest	4 miles, progression run	5 miles, general aerobic run	22 miles
5	3 miles, recovery run	4 miles, speed work: 1 mile, easy run with 3 × 20 sec strides to finish 4 × 400-m intervals with 400-m recovery jog 1 mile, cooldown Strength training	2 miles, run or walk	5 miles, general aerobic run with 3 × 20 sec strides to finish Strength training	Rest	6 miles, cutdown run: 1 mile, easy 4 miles, cutdown 1 mile, cooldown	8 miles, general aerobic run Strength training	28 miles

5K, 10K, and Half-Marathon Training Plans

Week	Mon	Tues	Wed	Thurs	Fri	Sat	Sun	Total
6	3 miles, recovery run	4 miles, speed work: 1 mile, easy run with 3 × 20 sec strides to finish 8 × 200-m repeats with 200-m recovery walk 1 mile, cooldown jog Strength training	3 miles, run or walk	5 miles, general aerobic run with 3 × 20 sec strides to finish Strength training	Rest	6 miles, cutdown run: 1 mile, easy run 4 miles, cutdown 1 mile, cooldown	8 miles, general aerobic run Strength training	29 miles
7 (recovery)	3 miles, recovery run	4 miles, speed work: 1 mile, easy run with 3 × 10 sec strides to finish 2 miles, sprint-floats for 10 × 100 m 1 mile, cooldown jog Strength training	3 miles, recovery run	3 miles, easy run with 3 × 20 sec strides to finish	Rest	3 miles, easy run with 3 × 20 sec strides to finish	5K test race: 1 mile, warm-up 5K, race pace 1 mile, cooldown	21.1 miles
8	3 miles, recovery run	5 miles, general aerobic run Strength training	3 miles, easy run	5 miles, speed work: 1 mile, easy run with 3 × 20 sec strides to finish 6 × 400-m intervals with 200-m recovery walk 1 mile, cooldown jog Strength training	Rest	7 miles, cutdown run: 1 mile, easy 5 miles, cutdown 1 mile, cooldown Strength training	9-10 miles, general aerobic run	32-33 miles

(continued)

Figure 9.4 Advanced 5K Training Plan *(continued)*

Week	Mon	Tues	Wed	Thurs	Fri	Sat	Sun	Total
9	3 miles, recovery run	4-5 miles, speed work: 1 mile, easy run with 3 × 20 sec strides to finish 8-10 × 200-m repeats with 200-m recovery walk 1 mile, cooldown jog Strength training	3 miles, easy run	4 miles, general aerobic run Strength training	Rest	5 miles, cutdown run: 1 mile, easy 3 miles, cutdown 1 mile, cooldown	5-7 miles, general aerobic run	24-27 miles
10 (taper)	3 miles, recovery run	4 miles, general aerobic run: 10 min, warm-up 8 × 1 min fast and 1 min recovery	Rest	3 miles, general aerobic run	Rest	3 miles, easy shakeout with 3 × 20 sec strides to finish	Race day!	13 miles + race

These plans assume that, from the start, you are able to finish a five- to six-mile run for the 5K plan and a seven- to nine-mile run for the 10K plan. You should be running 18 to 22 miles a week coming into the 5K plan and 25 to 28 miles per week coming into the 10K plan.

Figure 9.5 Advanced 10K Training Plan

Week	Mon	Tues	Wed	Thurs	Fri	Sat	Sun	Total
1	Rest	5 miles, hill circuits Strength training	3 miles, recovery run with 3 × 20 sec strides to finish	5 miles, cutdown run: 1 mile, easy 3 miles, cutdown 1 mile, cooldown	3 miles, recovery run	6 miles, race-pace run: 2 miles, aerobic pace 3 miles, goal race pace 2 miles, aerobic pace	7-8 miles, general aerobic run Strength training	29-30 miles

5K, 10K, and Half-Marathon Training Plans

Week	Mon	Tues	Wed	Thurs	Fri	Sat	Sun	Total
2	Rest	5 miles, hill circuits Strength training	3-4 miles, recovery run with 3 × 20 sec strides to finish	6 miles, cutdown run: 1 mile, easy 3 miles, cutdown 1 mile, cooldown	3 miles, recovery run	7 miles, race-pace run: 1 mile, aerobic pace 4 miles, goal race pace 2 miles, aerobic pace	8 miles, general aerobic run Strength training	32-33 miles
3	Rest	5-6 miles, speed work: 1 mile, easy run with 3 × 20 sec strides to finish 6-8 × 400-m intervals with 400-m recovery jog 1 mile, cooldown jog Strength training	4 miles, recovery run with 3 × 20 sec strides to finish	7 miles, cutdown run: 1 mile, easy 5 miles, cutdown 1 mile, cooldown	3 miles, recovery run	7 miles, race-pace run: 1 mile, aerobic pace 5 miles, goal race pace 1 mile, aerobic pace	9 miles, general aerobic run Strength training	35-36 miles
4 (recovery)	Rest	4 miles, speed work: 1 mile, easy 2 miles, sprint-floats for 8-10 × 100 m 1 mile, general aerobic run Strength training	3 miles, recovery run with 3 × 20 sec strides to finish	5 miles, general aerobic run Strength training	3 miles, recovery run	5 miles, race-pace run: 1 mile, aerobic pace 3 miles, goal race pace 1 mile, aerobic pace	5 miles, general aerobic run Strength training	25 miles
5	Rest	6-7 miles, speed work: 1 mile, easy run with 3 × 20 sec strides to finish 8-10 × 400-m intervals with 400-m recovery jog 1 mile, general aerobic run Strength training	4 miles, recovery run with 3 × 20 sec strides to finish	6 miles, cutdown run: 1 mile, easy 4 miles, cutdown 1 mile, cooldown Strength training	3 miles, recovery run	8 miles, race-pace run: 2 miles, aerobic pace 4 miles, goal race pace 2 miles, aerobic pace	10 miles, general aerobic run Strength training	37-38 miles

(continued)

Figure 9.5 Advanced 10K Training Plan *(continued)*

Week	Mon	Tues	Wed	Thurs	Fri	Sat	Sun	Total
6	Rest	5-6 miles, speed work: 1 mile, easy run with 3 × 20 sec strides to finish 8-9 × 600-m intervals with 600-m recovery jog 1 mile, general aerobic run Strength training	4 miles, recovery run with 3 × 20 sec strides to finish	7 miles, cutdown run: 1 mile, easy 5 miles, cutdown 1 mile, cooldown Strength training	3 miles, recovery run	8 miles, race-pace run: 2 miles, aerobic pace 4 miles, goal race pace 2 miles, aerobic pace	10 miles, general aerobic run Strength training	37-38 miles
7 (recovery)	Rest	4 miles, speed work: 1 mile, easy 3 miles, sprint-floats for 8-10 × 100 m 1 mile, general aerobic run Strength training	4 miles, recovery run	5 miles, easy run with 3 × 20 sec strides to finish	Rest	3 miles, easy run with 3 × 20 sec strides to finish	5K test race: 1 mile, warm-up 5K, race pace 1 mile, cooldown Strength training	21.1 miles
8	Rest	8 miles, speed work: 1 mile, easy run with 3 × 20 sec strides to finish 6 × 800-m intervals with 600-m easy recovery jog 1 mile, general aerobic run	4 miles, recovery run with 3 × 20 sec strides to finish	7 miles, cutdown run: 1 mile, easy 5 miles, cutdown 1 mile, cooldown Strength training	3 miles, recovery run	7 miles, race-pace run: 1 mile, aerobic pace 5 miles, goal race pace 1 mile, aerobic pace	10 miles, general aerobic run Strength training	39 miles

Week	Mon	Tues	Wed	Thurs	Fri	Sat	Sun	Total
				DAY				
9	Rest	5-6 miles, speed work: 1 mile, easy run with 3 × 20 sec strides to finish 8-10 × 400-m intervals with 200-m recovery jog 1 mile, cooldown jog Strength training	4 miles, recovery run	5-6 miles, general aerobic run	Rest	7 miles, cutdown run: 1 mile, easy 5 miles, cutdown 1 mile, cooldown with 3 × 20 sec strides to finish	5 miles, general aerobic run	26-28 miles
10 (taper)	Rest	4 miles, race-pace run: 1 mile, aerobic 2 miles, race pace 1 mile, aerobic	3 miles, easy run 8 × 100-m fast pick-ups and 100-m easy recovery jog	3 miles, easy run with 3 × 20 sec strides to finish	Rest	3 miles, easy shakeout with 3 × 20 sec strides to finish	Race day!	13 miles + race

Beginner and Intermediate Half-Marathon Training Plan

Before you move to the half-marathon distance, you should have some experience running for at least six months. This plan assumes that, at this stage, you can complete an 8- to 10-mile run and have maintained an average of 15 to 20 miles per week for the three months leading up to the beginning of your half-marathon training. In the plan provided (figure 9.6), you will see a range of distances given for each workout. For beginner half-marathoners, aim for the low end of the mileage range given; for intermediate half-marathoners, aim for the high end of the mileage range given.

Figure 9.6 Beginner and Intermediate Half-Marathon Training Plan

Week	Mon	Tues	Wed	Thurs	Fri	Sat	Sun	Total
1	Rest	4-6 miles, hilly fartleks Strength training	3 miles, recovery run with 3 × 20 sec strides to finish	4-6 miles, progression run (last 2 miles moderately fast)	Rest or 40-50 min cross-train	7-9 miles, general aerobic run Strength training	4 miles, recovery run	22-28 miles
2	Rest	5 miles, hill circuits Strength training	3 miles, recovery run with 3 × 20 sec strides to finish	5-7 miles, progression run (last 2-3 miles moderately fast)	Rest or 40-50 min cross-train	8-10 miles, general aerobic run Strength training	4 miles, recovery run	25-29 miles
3	Rest	5 miles, hill circuits Strength training	3 miles, recovery run with 3 × 20 sec strides to finish	6-8 miles, progression run (last 3-4 miles moderately fast)	Rest or 40-50 min cross-train	9-11 miles, general aerobic run Strength training	4 miles, recovery run	27-31 miles
4 (recovery)	Rest	4-5 miles, speed work: 1 mile, easy run with 3 × 20 sec strides to finish 2 miles, sprint-floats for 10-12 × 100 m 1 mile, general aerobic run Strength training	3 miles, recovery run with 3 × 20 sec strides to finish	5 miles, general aerobic run Strength training	Rest	5-7 miles, general aerobic run Strength training	3 miles, recovery run	20-23 miles

5K, 10K, and Half-Marathon Training Plans

Week	Mon	Tues	Wed	Thurs	Fri	Sat	Sun	Total
5	Rest	6-8 miles, speed work: 1 mile, easy run with 3 × 20 sec strides 8-10 × 400-m intervals with 400-m recovery jog 1 mile, cooldown jog Strength training	4 miles, recovery run with 3 × 20 sec strides to finish	6 miles, cutdown run: 1 mile, easy 4 miles, cutdown 1 mile, cooldown Strength training	Rest or 40-60 min cross-train	8-12 miles, general aerobic run Strength training	4 miles, recovery run	28-34 miles
6	Rest	6-8 miles, speed work: 1 mile, easy run with 3 × 20 sec strides 8-10 × 800-m intervals with 800-m recovery jog 1 mile, cooldown jog Strength training	4 miles, recovery run with 3 × 20 sec strides to finish	7 miles, cutdown run: 1 mile, easy 5 miles, cutdown 1 mile, cooldown Strength training	Rest or 40-60 min cross-train	10-12 miles, general aerobic run Strength training	5 miles, general aerobic run	32-36 miles
7 (recovery)	Rest	5-6 miles, general aerobic work: 1-2 miles, easy 2 miles, sprint-floats for 8-10 × 100 m 1-2 miles, general aerobic run Strength training	3 miles, recovery run with 3 × 20 sec strides to finish	6 miles, general aerobic run	Rest or 40-60 min cross-train	6-8 miles, progression run Strength training	3 miles, general aerobic run	23-26 miles

(continued)

Figure 9.6 Beginner and Intermediate Half-Marathon Training Plan *(continued)*

Week	Mon	Tues	Wed	Thurs	Fri	Sat	Sun	Total
8	Rest	7 miles, strength endurance work: 1 mile, easy 2 × 2 miles, 10K-15K race pace with 1 mile at aerobic recovery pace 1 mile, general aerobic run	3-4 miles, recovery run with 3 × 20 sec strides to finish	7-9 miles, cutdown run: 1 mile, easy 5-7 miles, cutdown 1 mile, cooldown Strength training	Rest or 40-60 min cross-train	11-13 miles, progression run Strength training	6 miles, recovery run	34-39 miles
9	Rest	6-8 miles, strength endurance work: 1 mile, easy 2-3 × 2 miles, 10K-15K race pace with 1 mile at aerobic recovery pace 1 mile, general aerobic run	4 miles, recovery run with 3 × 20 sec strides to finish	6 miles, general aerobic and speed work: 2 miles, easy 2 miles, sprint-floats for 8-10 × 100 m 2 miles, general aerobic run	3 miles, recovery run with 3 × 20 sec strides to finish	Rest or 40-60 min cross-train	7-9 miles, race-pace run: 2 miles, general aerobic run 4-6 miles, half-marathon pace 1 mile, easy	26-30 miles
10 (taper)	4 miles, race-pace run: 1 mile, general aerobic run 2 miles, race pace 1 mile, general aerobic run	Rest or 30 min cross-train	5 miles, taper and short speed work: 1 mile, general aerobic run 2 miles, sprint-floats for 5 × 100 m 1 mile, general aerobic run	3 miles, easy taper run with 3 × 20 sec strides to finish	Rest	3 miles, easy shakeout with 3 × 20 sec strides to finish	Race day!	15 miles + race

Chapter 10

Marathon and Ultramarathon Training Plans

The training plans provided here are for those looking to tackle a longer effort or race. There are plans for first-time marathoners and those who have some experience with the marathon distance. Generally, I recommend that first-time marathoners aim to finish feeling strong without necessarily setting a specific time goal. If this is your first marathon but you have a long race history, such as having run and raced many half-marathons, then setting some performance goals might be appropriate for you. As your training proceeds, you will likely have more information to determine general time goals that are helpful for devising a pacing plan for the race.

For the intermediate and advanced plans, you will see more targeted pace runs and speed workouts. Having some initial time goals based on your fitness at the beginning of the training cycle and your history of racing is appropriate, but you should fine-tune your goals as you progress through the training. The ultra plan presented here is for a 50K distance—likely your first 50K. While it's not necessary to have experience running marathons before taking on a 50K, it is a good idea. A lot can happen over the course of a marathon or a 50K, and having some experience solving problems on the go can be very useful.

As discussed earlier, always keep in mind that static programs do not respond to how you are feeling and reacting to the training. They do not adjust due to illness, unusual fatigue, or schedule interruptions. But you should monitor how you're feeling: Are you sleeping well? Is your resting heart rate steady? Is your heart rate where you expect it to be during workouts? Are you feeling unusually irritable? Are your normal paces feeling harder? If you experience any of the above for more than a few days, a recovery week might be warranted—or perhaps cutting out a recovery run that week for some extra rest. Addressing any lingering issues early is crucial for marathon and ultra training. The training can be fairly demanding, and everyone responds differently. Always listen to your body.

Marathon and Ultramarathon Training: General Terms and Recommendations

Before we get into the plans, there are some general recommendations and nomenclature you need to know that are specific to the marathon and ultramarathon training plans:

- Each day should begin with an easy dynamic warm-up (see exercises in chapter 8) followed by 10 minutes of easy running—no static stretching before running!
- Strides are fast, controlled accelerations. These are short and based on effort. Add in 20 seconds of jogging or walking between each acceleration. This is the only speed work included in the beginner plan.

- While there are no specific strength workouts prescribed in these plans, there are two principles to keep in mind: (1) Lift heavy—a weight you cannot lift for more than 8 to 12 repetitions or repeats. For a set, 2 to 3 × 8 to 12 repetitions of each exercise. (2) Hit the seven basic movement patterns: pull, press or push, carry, lunge, squat, rotation, and hinge.
- On the days you do a run and strength work, ideally you should do your run first—you are training for running, after all!—and then strength work after. It's best to do it several hours after your run, but if time doesn't permit this, do it when you can.
- General aerobic runs, the bulk of your training, should feel comfortable: run about 45 to 90 seconds per mile slower than your marathon pace. You should be able to carry on a conversation while running and not hear yourself breathing.
- Easy, or recovery, runs should be at a leisurely pace. You really can't run these too slow. Feel free to sing a song or walk if you feel like taking in a beautiful sunrise or sunset. You should feel better after the run than you did before.
- Hard-effort runs should feel like you're pushing beyond a comfortable pace. You will not be able to talk easily, and you will hear yourself breathing.
- Cutdown runs are a specific type of tempo run—a pace you can maintain for 60 minutes—that build faster as the run progresses. Begin at your aerobic pace, and run each mile 10 to 20 seconds faster than the previous mile. The aim is to work down to your goal race pace, or even a bit faster, by the final mile.
- Progression runs are done at a general aerobic pace for the first half or so and then at a slightly faster pace for the rest.
- Race-pace runs include a set number of miles at your goal race pace within a general aerobic run.
- Tempo runs begin and end with one mile at an easy aerobic pace. The tempo miles in between should be run between half-marathon pace and 10K pace—a pressing, uncomfortable pace but one you can maintain.
- Steady-state runs are still in the aerobic zone but are a bit faster, and your perceived effort is higher. This should be a slightly pressing pace—you can still talk, but not as easily, and you'll need to take breaths between sentences.
- Hill repeats are short (100 to 300 meters max) and are run on a moderately steep hill at a fast, pressing pace.
- Hill circuits are 200 to 800 meters long on a moderate hill. The number of repeats depends on the estimated length of the hill you use. This is how you perform a circuit:
    - Run strong up the hill—not a sprint, just a slightly pressing effort.
    - Jog for two to four minutes at the top.

(continued)

**Marathon and Ultramarathon Training Plans:
General Terms and Recommendations** *(continued)*

- Run down the hill quick and light.
- Jog for three to four minutes at the bottom.
- Run for 5 to 10 minutes at your general aerobic pace or until you reach the designated distance noted for the run.

- Hilly fartleks are performed by choosing a moderately hilly route and pushing some of the uphills faster as you feel like it. Do not sprint the hills—just run at a pushing pace.
- Hilly aerobic runs are done on a route with rolling hills or sustained climbs and descents. During the technical phase in the ultramarathon plan, focus on getting 75 to 100 percent of the total elevation gain and loss for your goal race over the course of each week. So, if your race has a net 5,000-foot gain and 5,000-foot loss, aim for around 5,000 feet of elevation gain and loss over the week. At a minimum, you should also do a couple runs per week on terrain that matches the technical demands of your goal race.
- Intervals are run at a hard pace but not an all-out effort—you should be able to get a word or two out (80 percent effort). You won't be fully recovered between faster segments.
- Repeats are run at a very hard effort, and you won't be able to talk (90 to 100 percent effort). The aim is complete recovery between harder bouts of running, but the faster segments are all-out efforts.
- Sprint-floats are a type of surge-and-glide run. These are best done on a 400-meter track; you sprint, or surge, on the 100-meter straightaway and float, or glide, around the turns. Run continuously and aim for an effort where you can maintain a consistent pace on the sprint segments for the entire workout without stopping to rest. Part of the challenge is to find a pace that is fast but not too fast. If your pace drops or your form begins breaking down, then this workout is done. If you don't have access to a track or it's difficult to get to, these can be done with a bit less precision on a flat road.
- With any speed work, you should end the workout when your form breaks down in any way or when your split time drops significantly.
- Taper runs use either a general aerobic or easy aerobic pace (noted in the plan). Remember, volume decreases but intensity remains steady during a taper.
- Regardless of the research, many runners prefer a cooldown of easier running to slowly back off after a hard effort, allowing their heart rate to lower and their breathing to settle. There seems to be at least a mental, if not a physiological, reason for a cooldown. Based on empirical observations, I often include an easier run to wrap up the workout.

Marathon Training Plans

First and foremost, I do not recommend jumping into marathon training without a sufficient aerobic base, so the beginner marathon training plan (figure 10.1) assumes you have been running somewhere around 20 to 25 miles a week for at least three months. The primary goal behind the beginner plan is to finish the race—it's not time specific, since you are presumably still a novice at this distance. The aim is to feel confident, healthy, and ready to run when you're standing on the starting line.

The intermediate and advanced plan (figure 10.2) is for runners who have run this distance before and are looking to run it faster or stronger, cut out walk breaks, or run a harder course. This plan assumes that, from the start, you are able to finish a 10-mile run. You should also be averaging at least 30 miles a week. In the plan provided, you will see a range of distances given for each workout; intermediate runners should aim for the low end of the mileage range given, while advanced runners should aim for the high end of the mileage range given.

Figure 10.1 Beginner Marathon Training Plan

Week	Mon	Tues	Wed	Thurs	Fri	Sat	Sun	Total
1	Rest	4-6 miles, general aerobic run; Strength training	3 miles, recovery run	4-6 miles, general aerobic run	Rest	9 miles, general aerobic run; Strength training	3 miles, recovery run	23-27 miles
2	Rest	4-6 miles, general aerobic run; Strength training	3 miles, recovery run	4-6 miles, general aerobic run	Rest	11 miles, general aerobic run; Strength training	4 miles, recovery run	26-30 miles
3	Rest	5-7 miles, general aerobic run; Strength training	3 miles, recovery run	5-7 miles, general aerobic run; Strength training	Rest	12 miles, general aerobic run; Strength training	5 miles, recovery run	30-34 miles
4 (recovery)	Rest	3-5 miles, general aerobic run; Strength training	2 miles, recovery run	3-5 miles, general aerobic run	Rest	7 miles, general aerobic run; Strength training	3 miles, recovery run	18-22 miles

(continued)

Figure 10.1 Beginner Marathon Training Plan *(continued)*

Week	Mon	Tues	Wed	Thurs	Fri	Sat	Sun	Total
5	Rest	6-7 miles, hilly aerobic run Strength training	3 miles, recovery run with 3 × 20 sec strides to finish	6-7 miles, general aerobic run	Rest	12 miles, medium aerobic run	5-7 miles, general aerobic run Strength training	32-36 miles
6	Rest	6-7 miles, hilly aerobic run Strength training	3 miles, recovery run with 3 × 20 sec strides to finish	6-7 miles, general aerobic run	Rest	14 miles, medium aerobic run	6-8 miles, general aerobic run Strength training	35-39 miles
7	Rest	7 miles, hilly fartlek Strength training	3 miles, recovery run with 3 × 20 sec strides to finish	6-8 miles, general aerobic run	Rest	15 miles, medium aerobic run	7-9 miles, general aerobic run Strength training	38-42 miles
8 (recovery)	Rest	4-6 miles, general aerobic run	2 miles, recovery run	4-6 miles, general aerobic run	Rest	9 miles, general aerobic run Strength training	4 miles, recovery run	23-27 miles
9	Rest	6-8 miles, general aerobic run Strength training	4 miles, recovery run with 3 × 20 sec strides to finish	6-8 miles, tempo run with 1-mile warm-up	Rest	14 miles, progression run (last 4 miles at pressing pace)	7-9 miles, general aerobic run Strength training	37-43 miles
10	Rest	7-8 miles, general aerobic run	4 miles, recovery run with 3 × 20 sec strides to finish	7-8 miles, tempo run with 1-mile warm-up	Rest	15 miles, medium aerobic run	8-10 miles, general aerobic run Strength training	41-45 miles
11	Rest	6-8 miles, general aerobic run Strength training	4 miles, recovery run with 3 × 20 sec strides to finish	7-8 miles, tempo run with 1-mile warm-up	Rest	15 miles, progression run (last 5 miles at pressing pace)	8-10 miles, general aerobic run Strength training	40-45 miles

Marathon and Ultramarathon Training Plans

Week	DAY								Total
	Mon	Tues	Wed	Thurs	Fri	Sat	Sun	
12 (recovery)	Rest	5 miles, general aerobic run	3 miles, recovery run with 3 × 20 sec strides to finish	5 miles, general aerobic run	Rest	8 miles, medium aerobic run Strength training	5 miles, general aerobic run	26 miles
13	Rest	6-8 miles, general aerobic run Strength training	4 miles, recovery run with 3 × 20 sec strides to finish	6-8 miles, general aerobic run: 1 mile aerobic warmup with 2-3 × 10 sec strides to finish 3-4 × 800 m at pressing pace 800-m aerobic recovery jog Finish remaining miles at general aerobic pace	Rest	16 miles, progression run (last 5 miles at pressing pace)	10 miles, general aerobic run Strength training	42-46 miles
14	Rest	6-8 miles, general aerobic run Strength training	4 miles, recovery run with 3 × 20 sec strides to finish	6-8 miles, general aerobic run: 1 mile, aerobic warmup with 2-3 × 10 sec strides to finish 4-5 × 800 m at pressing pace 800-m aerobic recovery jog Finish remaining miles at general aerobic pace	Rest	18 miles, long aerobic run	10 miles, general aerobic run Strength training	44-48 miles

(continued)

Figure 10.1 Beginner Marathon Training Plan *(continued)*

Week	Mon	Tues	Wed	Thurs	Fri	Sat	Sun	Total
15	Rest	6-8 miles, general aerobic run Strength training	4 miles, recovery	7-9 miles, general aerobic run: 1 mile, aerobic warmup with 2-3 × 10 sec strides to finish 6-7 × 800 m at pressing pace 800-m aerobic recovery jog Finish remaining miles at general aerobic pace	Rest	16 miles, long aerobic run	12 miles, progression run (last 5 miles at pressing pace) Strength training	45-49 miles
16 (taper)	Rest	7 miles, general aerobic run Strength training	4 miles, recovery run with 3 × 20 sec strides to finish	5-6 miles, general aerobic run: 1 mile, aerobic warmup 12 × 100 m at pressing pace 100-m aerobic recovery jog Finish remaining miles at general aerobic pace	Rest	12 miles, medium aerobic run	5-7 miles, general aerobic run Strength training	33-36 miles

Week	Mon	Tues	Wed	Thurs	Fri	Sat	Sun	Total
17 (taper)	Rest	5-6 miles, general aerobic run Strength training	4 miles, recovery run	5-6 miles, general aerobic run: 1 mile, aerobic warmup 8 × 100 m at pressing pace 100-m aerobic recovery jog Finish remaining miles at general aerobic pace	Rest	8 miles, medium aerobic run	4 miles, general aerobic run	26-28 miles
18 (taper)	Rest	4 miles, taper run: 1 mile, general aerobic pace 2 miles, marathon pace 1 mile, general aerobic pace	3 miles, general aerobic run: 1 mile, aerobic warmup 5 × 100-m fast pickups 100-m easy recovery jog	3 miles, easy taper run with 3 × 20 sec strides to finish	Rest	3 miles, easy shakeout with 3 × 20 sec strides to finish	Race day!	13 miles + race

Figure 10.2 Intermediate and Advanced Marathon Training Plan

Week	Mon	Tues	Wed	Thurs	Fri	Sat	Sun	Total
1	Rest	5-7 miles, general aerobic run Strength training	4 miles, recovery run	5-7 miles, general aerobic run	Rest	10 miles, general aerobic run Strength training	5 miles, recovery run	29-33 miles
2	Rest	5-7 miles, general aerobic run Strength training	4 miles, recovery run	5-7 miles, general aerobic run	Rest	12 miles, general aerobic run Strength training	5 miles, recovery run	31-35 miles

(continued)

Figure 10.2 Intermediate and Advanced Marathon Training Plan *(continued)*

Week	Mon	Tues	Wed	Thurs	Fri	Sat	Sun	Total
3	Rest	6-8 miles, general aerobic run Strength training	4 miles, recovery run	6-8 miles, general aerobic run	Rest	13 miles, general aerobic run Strength training	7 miles, recovery run	36-40 miles
4 (recovery)	Rest	4-6 miles, general aerobic run	3 miles, recovery run	4-6 miles, general aerobic run	Rest	8 miles, general aerobic run Strength training	4 miles, recovery run	23-27 miles
5	Rest	7-9 miles, hill circuits Strength training	4 miles, recovery run with 3 × 20 sec strides to finish	7-9 miles, general aerobic run	4 miles, recovery run with 3 × 20 sec strides to finish	6-8 miles, cutdown run: 1 mile, easy 4-6 miles, cutdown 1 mile, cooldown	13 miles, medium aerobic run Strength training	41-47 miles
6	Rest	7-9 miles, hill circuits Strength training	4 miles, recovery run with 3 × 20 sec strides to finish	7-9 miles, general aerobic run	4 miles, recovery run with 3 × 20 sec strides to finish	7-9 miles, cutdown run: 1 mile, easy 5-7 miles, cutdown 1 mile, cooldown	14 miles, medium aerobic run Strength training	43-49 miles
7	Rest	7-8 miles, hill circuits Strength training	4 miles, recovery run with 3 × 20 sec strides to finish	7-8 miles, general aerobic run	4 miles, recovery run with 3 × 20 sec strides to finish	14 miles, marathon-pace run: 2 miles, aerobic pace 10 miles, marathon pace 2 miles, aerobic pace	5-6 miles, general aerobic run Strength training	41-44 miles
8 (recovery)	Rest	4-6 miles, general aerobic run	2 miles, recovery run	4-6 miles, general aerobic run	4 miles, recovery run with 3 × 20 sec strides to finish	10 miles, general aerobic run Strength training	5 miles, recovery run	29-33 miles

Marathon and Ultramarathon Training Plans

Week	Mon	Tues	Wed	Thurs	Fri	Sat	Sun	Total
9	Rest	7-9 miles, strength endurance work: 1 mile, easy 2-3 × 2 miles, 10K-15K race pace with 1 mile at aerobic recovery pace 1 mile, general aerobic run Strength training	4 miles, recovery run with 3 × 20 sec strides to finish	7-9 miles, general aerobic run	4 miles, recovery run with 3 × 20 sec strides to finish	8-10 miles, cutdown run: 1 mile, easy 6-8 miles, cutdown 1 mile, cooldown	14 miles, medium aerobic run Strength training	44-50 miles
10	Rest	7-9 miles, strength endurance work: 1 mile, easy 2-3 × 2 miles, 10K-15K race pace with 1 mile at aerobic recovery pace 1 mile, general aerobic run Strength training	4 miles, recovery run with 3 × 20 sec strides to finish	7-9 miles, general aerobic run	4 miles, recovery run with 3 × 20 sec strides to finish	9-11 miles, cutdown run: 1 mile, easy 7-9 miles, cutdown 1 mile, cooldown	16 miles, general aerobic run Strength training	47-53 miles
11	Rest	7-8 miles, cutdown run: 1 mile, easy 5-6 miles, cutdown 1 mile, cooldown Strength training	4 miles, recovery run with 3 × 20 sec strides to finish	9 miles, general aerobic run	4 miles, recovery run with 3 × 20 sec strides to finish	Half-marathon training race: 1 mile, warm-up 13.1 miles, marathon race pace 1 mile, easy aerobic run	7-8 miles, general aerobic run Strength training	46.1-48.1 miles

(continued)

Figure 10.2 Intermediate and Advanced Marathon Training Plan *(continued)*

Week	Mon	Tues	Wed	Thurs	Fri	Sat	Sun	Total
12 (recovery)	Rest	5-7 miles, general aerobic run	4 miles, recovery run with 3 × 20 sec strides to finish	5-7 miles, general aerobic run	4 miles recovery run with 3 × 20 sec strides to finish	10 miles, medium aerobic run	7 miles, general aerobic run Strength training	35-39 miles
13	Rest	8-10 miles, general aerobic run Strength training	4 miles, recovery run with 3 × 20 sec strides to finish	6-8 miles, general aerobic run and speed work: 1 mile, aerobic warmup with 2-3 × 10 sec strides to finish 3 × 800 m at pressing pace 800-m recovery jog 1 mile, aerobic pace	4 miles, recovery run with 3 × 20 sec strides to finish	10-12 miles, cutdown run: 1 mile, easy 8-10 miles, cutdown 1 mile, cooldown	17 miles, long aerobic run Strength training	49-55 miles
14	Rest	8-10 miles, general aerobic run Strength training	4 miles, recovery run with 3 × 20 sec strides to finish	6-8 miles, general aerobic run: 1-2 miles, aerobic pace with 2-3 × 10 sec strides to finish 4 × 800 m at pressing pace 800-m recovery jog 1 mile, aerobic pace	4 miles, recovery run with 3 × 20 sec strides to finish	10-12 miles, cutdown run: 1 mile, easy 8-10 miles, cutdown 1 mile, cooldown	18 miles, long aerobic run Strength training	50-56 miles

Marathon and Ultramarathon Training Plans

Week	Mon	Tues	Wed	Thurs	Fri	Sat	Sun	Total
15	Rest	6-8 miles, general aerobic run Strength training	4 miles, recovery run	7-9 miles, general aerobic run: 1-2 miles, aerobic pace with 2-3 × 10 sec strides to finish 5 × 800 m at marathon pace 800-m recovery jog 1 mile, aerobic pace	Rest	18 miles, long aerobic run: 16 miles, marathon pace 1 mile, aerobic pace 14 miles, marathon pace 1 mile, aerobic pace	10 miles, general aerobic run Strength training	45-49 miles
16 (taper)	Rest	6-8 miles, general aerobic run	4 miles, recovery run with 3 × 20 sec strides to finish	5-6 miles, general aerobic pace and speed work: 1-2 miles, general aerobic pace 2 miles, sprint-floats for 8-10 × 100 m 1-2 miles, general aerobic pace	Rest	15 miles, long aerobic run	5-7 miles, general aerobic run	35-40 miles

(continued)

Figure 10.2 Intermediate and Advanced Marathon Training Plan *(continued)*

Week	Mon	Tues	Wed	Thurs	Fri	Sat	Sun	Total
17	Rest	5-7 miles, general aerobic run	4 miles, recovery run	5-6 miles, general aerobic pace and speed work: 1-2 miles, general aerobic pace 2 miles, sprint-float at 8-10 × 100m 1-2 miles, general aerobic pace	Rest	5K tune-up race: 2 miles, warm-up 5K at 10K pace 2 miles, easy cooldown	5 miles, general aerobic run	26.1-29.1 miles
18	Rest	5 miles, marathon-pace taper run: 1 mile, easy aerobic 2 miles, race pace 2 miles, easy aerobic	3 miles, easy aerobic taper run: 8 × 100-m fast pick-ups and 100-m recovery jog	3 miles, easy aerobic taper run with 3 × 20 sec strides to finish	Rest	3 miles, easy shakeout with 3 × 20 sec strides to finish	Race day!	14 miles + race

Ultramarathon Training Plan

An ultramarathon is, by definition, anything longer than the marathon distance. Generally, ultras range from 50K to 200 miles or more, with 50K to 100 miles being the most popular options.

Ultras come in many forms—road, gravel, track, and trail (or a combination)—and vary greatly concerning their technical demands (rocks, roots, slickrock, sand, etc.) and elevation gain and loss (how much climbing and descending is involved). As trail running becomes more popular, many shorter distances are added into the mix. For trail races in general, it's important in training to focus on course-specific demands, especially concerning elevation and technical aspects. The optimal time for race-specific training is as you get closer to the race, so fewer race-specific adaptations appear earlier in the training cycle. For this reason, it's difficult to provide a general training plan for all ultras or trail races.

The plan provided here is for a trail race with moderate elevation gain or loss and some technical running (figure 10.3). For flatter, nontechnical races, you can still follow this plan—but during the last phase of training, focus on different race-specific runs. You likely won't need to focus on technical aspects or elevation, but the volume recommendations remain the same.

Figure 10.3 Ultramarathon Training Plan

Week	Mon	Tues	Wed	Thurs	Fri	Sat	Sun	Total
1	Rest	7-8 miles, general aerobic run	5 miles, recovery run	7-8 miles, general aerobic run	5 miles, recovery run	10 miles, general aerobic run Strength training	5 miles, recovery run	39-41 miles
2	Rest	7-8 miles, general aerobic run Strength training	5 miles, recovery run	7-8 miles, general aerobic run	5 miles, recovery run	12 miles, general aerobic run Strength training	6 miles, recovery run	42-44 miles
3	Rest	7-8 miles, general aerobic run Strength training	4 miles, recovery run	7-8 miles, general aerobic run Strength training	4 miles, recovery run	13 miles, general aerobic run Strength training	7 miles, recovery run	42-44 miles
4 (recovery)	Rest	5-6 miles, general aerobic run	3 miles, recovery run	5-6 miles, general aerobic run	Rest	9 miles, general aerobic run Strength training	4 miles, recovery run	26-28 miles
5	Rest	8-9 miles, hill circuits Strength training	4 miles, recovery run with 3 × 20 sec strides to finish	6-8 miles, cutdown run: 1 mile, easy 4-6 miles, cutdown 1 mile, cooldown	4 miles, recovery run with 3 × 20 sec strides to finish	14 miles, progression run (last 5 miles at pressing pace)	10 miles, medium aerobic run Strength training	46-49 miles

(continued)

Figure 10.3 Ultramarathon Training Plan *(continued)*

Week	Mon	Tues	Wed	Thurs	Fri	Sat	Sun	Total
6	Rest	7-9 miles, hill circuits Strength training	4 miles, recovery run with 3 × 20 sec strides to finish	7-9 miles, cutdown run: 1 mile, easy 5-7 miles, cutdown 1 mile, cooldown	4 miles, recovery run with 3 × 20 sec strides to finish	15 miles, medium aerobic run	14 miles, medium aerobic run Strength training	51-55 miles
7	Rest	7-9 miles, hill circuits Strength training	4 miles, recovery run with 3 × 20 sec strides to finish	8-10 miles, cutdown run: 1 mile, easy 6-8 miles, cutdown 1 mile, cooldown	4 miles, recovery run with 3 × 20 sec strides to finish	15 miles, progression run (last 5 miles at pressing pace)	5-6 miles, general aerobic run Strength training	43-48 miles
8 (recovery)	Rest	6-7 miles, general aerobic run Strength training	4 miles, recovery run with 3 × 20 sec strides to finish	6-7 miles, general aerobic run	4 miles, recovery run with 3 × 20 sec strides to finish	12 miles, general aerobic run	6 miles, recovery run Strength training	38-40 miles
9	Rest	8-10 miles, general aerobic run Strength training	4 miles, recovery run with 3 × 20 sec strides to finish	8-10 miles, cutdown run: 1 mile, easy 6-8 miles, cutdown 1 mile, cooldown	4 miles, recovery run with 3 × 20 sec strides to finish	16 miles, progression run (last 5 miles at pressing pace)	14 miles, medium aerobic run Strength training	54-58 miles
10	Rest	6-8 miles, general aerobic run Strength training	4 miles, recovery run with 3 × 20 sec strides to finish	10-12 miles, cutdown run: 1 mile, easy 8-10 miles, cutdown 1 mile, cooldown	4 miles, recovery run with 3 × 20 sec strides to finish	18 miles, medium aerobic run	14 miles, general aerobic run Strength training	56-60 miles

Marathon and Ultramarathon Training Plans

	DAY							
Week	Mon	Tues	Wed	Thurs	Fri	Sat	Sun	Total
11	Rest	6-8 miles, general aerobic run Strength training	4 miles, recovery run with 3 × 20 sec strides to finish	7-8 miles, cutdown run: 1 mile, easy 5-6 miles, cutdown 1 mile, cooldown	4 miles, recovery run with 3 × 20 sec strides to finish	25-26 miles, long aerobic run	5-7 miles, general aerobic run Strength training	51-57 miles
12 (recovery)	Active rest: 20 min, walk, bike, or swim	5-7 miles, general aerobic run	4 miles, recovery run with 3 × 20 sec strides to finish	5-7 miles, general aerobic run	4 miles, recovery run with 3 × 20 sec strides to finish	10 miles, medium aerobic run	7 miles, general aerobic run Strength training	35-39 miles + 20 min
13 (technical phase: aim for 75%-100% net race elevation gain or loss over the week)	Rest	8-10 miles, hilly aerobic run Strength training	4 miles, recovery run with 3 × 20 sec strides to finish	8-10 miles, hilly aerobic run	4 miles, recovery run with 3 × 20 sec strides to finish	18 miles, trail run	15 miles, general aerobic run Strength training	57-61 miles
14 (technical phase: aim for 75%-100% net race elevation gain or loss over the week)	Rest	8-10 miles, hilly aerobic run Strength training	4 miles, recovery run with 3 × 20 sec strides to finish	8-10 miles, hilly aerobic run	4 miles, recovery run with 3 × 20 sec strides to finish	20 miles, trail run	12 miles, general aerobic run Strength training	56-60 miles
15 (technical phase: aim for 75%-100% net race elevation gain or loss over the week)	Rest	8-10 miles, hilly aerobic run Strength training	4 miles, recovery run	8-10 miles, hilly aerobic run	4 miles, recovery run	18 miles, trail run	14 miles, medium aerobic run Strength training	56-60 miles

(continued)

Figure 10.3 Ultramarathon Training Plan *(continued)*

Week	Mon	Tues	Wed	Thurs	Fri	Sat	Sun	Total
16 (taper)	Rest	6-8 miles, general aerobic run Strength training	4 miles, recovery run with 3 × 20 sec strides to finish	6-8 miles, general aerobic run	Rest	15 miles, long aerobic run	5-7 miles, general aerobic run Strength training	36-42 miles
17 (taper)	Rest	6-7 miles, general aerobic run	4 miles, recovery run	6-7 miles, general aerobic run Strength training	Rest	8-10 miles, medium aerobic run	5 miles, general aerobic run	29-33 miles
18 (taper)	Rest	5 miles, general aerobic run	Rest	4 miles, easy taper run with 3 × 20 sec strides to finish	Rest	3 miles, easy shakeout with 3 × 20 sec strides to finish	Race day!	12 miles + race

Chapter 11

Transitional Training Plans

With traditional training plans, a macrocycle is often broken up into three segments, or mesocycles—preparation, competition, and transition or offseason—as you learned in chapter 4. There are two types of transition periods: (1) a recovery or detraining cycle and (2) an out-of-season cycle, or what I call a *shoulder season*, to focus on supporting skills such as strength or speed. Both allow you to reset and refresh your mind and body so you can continue to build on your previous training.

Recovery or Detraining Cycle

When you're training for a goal, your training is broken up into mesocycles that focus on specific adaptations—endurance, strength, speed, lactate threshold, etc. After a dedicated training cycle, a recovery or detraining mesocycle should follow to allow your body and mind to recover from the training and from reaching your goal. This recovery or detraining mesocycle can come in two general varieties: (1) a recovery period of lighter workouts, depending on the length and demands of the goal reached or (2) a detraining period that is a purposeful time of rest and rebuilding for both mind and body.

Let's assume you just accomplished a challenging goal and now feel the need for a break, or after training hard for a period of time, you need some downtime to recharge your physical and mental batteries. Having a recovery or detraining period is an important aspect of training that you must anticipate and schedule into your annual plan.

Recovery Plan

Recovery time after running a race or reaching a goal can vary depending on several factors, including the distance of the race or goal, your fitness level and experience with the distance, and how hard you pushed yourself. Here are some general guidelines:

- *Short-term goals and short-distance races (5K and under):* Recovery time may be fairly short, typically a day or two of easy active recovery (walking, cycling, swimming, or yoga) before returning to normal training.
- *Medium goals and middle-distance races (10K to half-marathon):* It might take a few days to a week of active recovery (walking, jogging, cycling, swimming, or yoga). It's essential to focus on rest, hydration, nutrition, and good sleep during this time.
- *Long-term goals and long-distance races (marathon, ultramarathon, or a goal over 20 miles):* Recovery can take several weeks. Your body will need time to repair muscles and allow for adaptations.

Why do I emphasize active recovery rather than complete rest? Active recovery brings healing blood and, with it, nutrients to your muscles, tendons, and ligaments while also maintaining joint mobility and ROM. It also has mental benefits, keeping you moving and doing activities you enjoy. To give you an idea of what a recovery plan might look like following a marathon, 50K, or even a half-marathon, look at figure 11.1.

Figure 11.1 Sample Recovery Plan Following a Half-Marathon, Marathon, or 50K

Week	Mon	Tues	Wed	Thurs	Fri	Sat	Sun	Total
1	Active rest: 20 min, walk, easy spin, or swim	Active rest: 20 min, walk, easy spin, or swim	30 min, easy jog	Rest	40 min, easy jog	Rest	3 miles, recovery run	3 miles + 110 min
2	Rest	3 miles, recovery run	30 min, easy jog	3 miles, recovery run	Rest	5 miles, recovery run Strength training	3 miles, recovery run	14 miles + 30 min
3	Rest	5 miles, recovery run	3 miles, recovery run	5 miles, recovery run with 3 × 20 sec strides to finish Strength training	Rest	7 miles, recovery run Strength training	5 miles, recovery run	25 miles
4	Rest	6 miles, general aerobic run Strength training	3 miles, recovery run with 3 × 20 sec strides to finish	6 miles, general aerobic run Strength training	Rest	8 miles, medium aerobic run	6 miles, general aerobic run Strength training	29 miles

Deloading or Detraining Plan

Detraining, or deloading, is defined as a reduction of focused training for specific adaptations brought about by that training (Bosquet and Mujika 2012). Basically, you're just taking a break from intense training, whatever that looks like for you. Training volume, frequency, and intensity all decrease, reducing both physical and mental stress. It lasts longer than a recovery week or two but is short enough that you don't lose too much fitness and have to start from scratch. Research shows that within the first couple weeks of detraining, very little fitness is lost (this is also true for injuries, which is one reason to address injuries quickly). But after two weeks, fitness drops precipitously, so you want to keep the deloading phase long enough to reap the benefits without extending it so long you lose too much base fitness.

The chronic stress of training adds up over time, and there's a chance that after a certain point, adaptations slow down. Taking a break reduces this chronic stress so that when you return to training, your body will respond better to the stress applied. This is also why you change focus during different training phases.

But this isn't just about physical stress; it's also about mental stress. The deloading phase is planned and intentional. When you make your annual plan, you should include a deloading cycle. This is not downtime caused by injury, illness, or life stresses. Why? This time needs to be a choice if you are going to reap the mental benefits from a reduction in training; dealing with life interruptions due to things out of your control rarely leads to mental rebuilding. These interruptions often only add to mental angst and frustration. A time of deloading is something you embrace because it's good for you in the long run. This is part of a well-planned training program. Detraining is not the absence of training—it *is* training. This is a time to reset your mind and body. Schedule these breaks into your annual plan.

Of course, understanding how to organize this deloading period is important for a robust recovery without significant fitness loss. When done well, the deloading cycle will allow you to recover well without losing the fitness you've worked so hard to build. A four-week cycle optimizes this process of deloading and then rebuilding. The goal is to come back feeling physically and mentally recharged and ready to get back to structured training. These rest periods ideally leave you eager to get back to running.

The best organization for these weeks will look something like the following:

Week One

Do no exercise, or do only easy cross-training. For runners, that means *no running*. Instead, do some easy swimming, cycling, or walking based on what you feel like doing. This first deloading week is important for recovery and sets the stage for your next training cycle.

Week Two

Add in two to three short, easy runs. Maybe throw in a relaxing swim or spin. This needs to stay short and easy. This is a great time to do other things—go for a nice walk or hike, explore a new area, and get out of your routine.

Week Three

Start building things back, but with lower volume and intensity. At this point, aim for 40 to 60 percent of the volume and 30 to 60 percent of the intensity you were doing in training. For example, if you were running 30 miles a week, aim for 10 to 18 miles this week. Frequency will be less than what you were doing at peak training, but start moving toward a maintenance volume. If you were running six days a week, now aim for about four days a week, perhaps adding in some cross-training one or two days a week. If you ran 40 miles a week during peak training, your goal at this point is 25 to 30 miles. If you were doing two high-intensity runs a week, add one back in, but it will be a bit shorter and at a slightly lower intensity.

Week Four

At this point, you should be moving back up to a maintenance level as you build back your base. If you've done well the last three weeks, you feel a bit antsy to get back to running. These breaks, ideally, bring you to a point where you can't wait to get back into your running routine. You likely feel fresh and recharged.

Inevitably, I will have a runner come to me after sustaining an injury and enduring the resulting time off to heal and rehab, and they believe this counts as a detraining period. Unfortunately, that's not the case. A detraining period must be intentional, not something forced on you. Again, this is not about healing but rather about unloading both mind and body. Healing and rehabbing an injury doesn't fulfill this purpose because it isn't something you choose, and it's often something you wish wasn't happening. A deloading period is something to look forward to as a time of well-earned rest and recharge.

It's important that you buy into the whole idea of this essential part of training. If you have a hard time pulling back and feel anxious and uneasy for these four weeks, then the benefits will not be as obvious. Physically, you may be ready to get back at it, but mentally, the stress of the previous four weeks will undermine the benefits of the recharge. If this is you, this might be an opportunity to really examine your feelings about running, self-identity, and self-value.

As a coach, I've noticed that athletes often welcome these downtimes when they coincide with other demands in their lives. Some prefer time off during certain holidays or when the weather is particularly cold or hot. Some want time off during heavy work periods or when their children are either in or out of school. Whatever your preferences, plan your breaks and your goals for times that work for you. For example, if fall is your favorite time to run, scheduling a break during this time will only frustrate you as you spend your days wishing you were out there running. However, if there is a goal you really want to pursue that may not fit into your normal life flow, but you understand that and are still willing to make the commitment, which means that other things may need to be adjusted, then that's okay—if you recognize and accept the consequences of your choices.

Out-of-Season Cycle or Shoulder Season

Let's suppose you just ran a marathon. It's October, and you have another marathon planned for the spring. You've taken a few weeks to recover, and now you're trying to figure out what to do for the next month or two. You don't need to focus specifically on marathon training yet, so what can you do now to build on your fitness and address some possible weaknesses so that you go into the next marathon training cycle stronger? Or let's suppose you just raced your first 5K. Now you want to do some more 5Ks, and maybe you want to race them faster; you want to see just how fast you can run a 5K. Are there things you can do during this training lull to make yourself a better, more well-rounded runner?

A shoulder season allows you to work on your weaknesses. In many cases, you select what you think you're good at based on your previous experiences. You usually prefer doing the things you're good at because that makes you feel good and avoid doing the things you believe you aren't so good at because they make you feel weaker or slower. Working on your weaknesses can feel frustrating and uncomfortable, but sometimes it's beneficial. While it's good to use your strengths, you often improve the most by focusing on your weaknesses.

The problem here is that it's rather unpleasant to work on things you're not good at. I'd much rather go for a cruising 20-mile run than do six 800-meter repeats at 3K to 5K pace. I dread 800-meter repeats. Why? I'm just not that good at them, and they hurt. But at some point, when you really desire to push yourself, to see how fast you can run a particular distance, to beat or best yourself, you must acknowledge that it is probably your weaknesses, not your strengths, that make the crucial difference.

These shoulder seasons offer you an opportunity to get uncomfortable and work on your weaknesses. Now is the time to reflect on your training and see where you tend to focus.

As a coach, I can often look at a runner's race times and see where their natural talents lie. Take a runner who runs a half-marathon at about the same pace as a 5K—maybe a little faster for the 5K, but not significantly. This runner would benefit from adding some short speed work. Likewise, a runner who races a fast 5K but gets severely fatigued eight miles into a half-marathon likely needs to introduce long runs, tempo runs, and maybe more weekly mileage.

You can also ask yourself, "What do I find more enjoyable, and what seems to come easier to me? What do I tend to avoid?" If an upcoming workout causes an increase in anticipatory stress, it's probably something you need to work on and become more comfortable with. If you stick with it—through the challenges of feeling slow or weak or somehow not measuring up—you will likely reap huge benefits, and you may even start to enjoy what you once avoided. Put your ego aside and welcome this uncomfortable challenge. It will allow you to bring newly developed fitness into the next training cycle. Depending on your goals, you could use another training program provided here to help focus your intermediate goals. As an example, if you wish to improve your half-marathon or marathon performance, you could use an intermediate or advanced 5K or 10K plan between focused half-marathon or marathon training cycles.

All-comers meets are another option that can be a lot of fun for those looking for more social connection and fun competition. Many towns offer these, especially during the summer months, where you can drop in and race different distances. Parkruns, traditionally popular in the UK, are also becoming more popular around the world. These are often fun cross-country-style races or short road races. These options can be fun to focus on for a short time to increase speed without the type of training and emotional commitment that a larger goal often entails.

Perhaps you want to try a short triathlon or a relay race such as Ragnar. Or perhaps you want to see if a local running group is right for you. These, too, will introduce different training stresses, environments, and opportunities to learn new things while also connecting with different people.

It's important in a shoulder season to embrace novel activities, things you might not normally do, but also to surprise your body and mind. Keep things fresh. Spice things up. Make an effort to run with others more or to try something you've never done before. It's easy to get stuck in a rut, and during training, those habits of consistency are important, but stirring things up occasionally is also important physically, mentally, and even socially—meeting new people who do different things.

While running is a mostly linear activity, training for running needn't be linear. There are ebbs and flows over months and years of running. There are so many opportunities to sample new challenges. These options are not limited by age but are driven by the desire to pursue things you enjoy or are motivated to explore. For many runners, the ultimate goal is to keep running for life. You have ample examples now of those who are doing just that—running into their 70s, 80s, 90s, and even 100s! Taking care of your body through smart training, good nutrition and sleep habits, and an annual recharge will help keep you able to pursue your goals for the long run. There are times when less is more, and welcoming those phases is just as important as any other part of training—fitness, competition, personal challenge, and running for life, which will offer seemingly unlimited options.

PART IV

COMPETING

Chapter 12

Preparing to Compete

For some runners, racing is an integral part of running. For others, racing isn't really a part of their running practice. It's similar to how many approach yoga—running can become a daily personal practice, something you enjoy and make a part of your daily life to stay physically and mentally healthy. As I mentioned earlier, I ran for years and only occasionally jumped into a race for fun. But my practice of running is just a part of my day and has taken me places, on foot, that I might not have seen otherwise. Year in and year out, I watch the seasons change. While traveling, I see new places in a more intimate way, running through cities and towns and down country roads, getting a feel for a new place. The daily practice of running is my time to be present in the world and in my life.

However, I have also spent years focusing on training for races that mattered to me for personal reasons. I've run in places I might never have seen. I've made countless new friends at races, many of whom remain close. And racing encourages me to push myself and test my limits, both on the racecourse and during training. That changes me for the better.

Why Race?

Racing can be a motivating and fun way to challenge yourself, meet new people, spend time with running friends, and see new places. Racing challenges you to push yourself beyond your comfort zone, whether that concerns time or distance or the race itself. Every race teaches you something about yourself. Sometimes the lessons are hard. Sometimes what you learn is uplifting. Sometimes you discover you're stronger and tougher than you think. Sometimes you discover things you can work on. Sometimes racing can be fun, and sometimes it can hurt.

Perhaps you are feeling a bit reluctant, or nervous, to sign up for a race. Here are some reasons I often hear:

I'm not a competitive person.

Maybe you don't see yourself as competitive but believe that it's a necessary part of racing. I've heard this claim from a lot of runners 50 and over, and I usually accept it at face value but also believe there might be something going on beneath the surface. Sometimes you feel uncomfortable putting yourself out there for all to see. Sometimes you worry about judgment from others and even yourself. And sometimes you believe that being competitive is a negative attribute. I find that women in particular offer this as a reason for not racing. For many women, being competitive is seen as aggressive and can stir up gender stereotypes. But is there really anything aggressive about challenging yourself?

I don't see myself as an athlete.

I hear so many runners say they aren't real runners or athletes. Why? Perhaps you have this idea that being a real runner requires you to run a certain distance or pace—or you must have been doing it all your life or must achieve a certain number of races, and on and on. Perhaps you've felt, or are feeling, like an impostor. You know the saying that comparison is the thief of joy, and you understand the veracity of that claim, yet you still compare—you compare yourself to others, to your younger self, and to the ideas you have about what you should be doing or should be able to do. You allow self-doubt to creep in. You deflect anticipated judgment through self-deprecation. Social media doesn't help because you see so many others doing incredible things you can only dream of.

But here's the thing: If you run, you are a real runner—and you can even walk. You can run and walk. You can walk and run. You can run and get tired and stop and go home. You can try again tomorrow. The only thing that matters—the only thing that makes you a runner and an athlete—is that you keep at it. You try. Sometimes you succeed, and sometimes you don't. But each time you try, that makes all the difference in your life. So, keep trying. That's what makes you an athlete. Think about your strengths at work or with your family or friends and bring those to your runs. At the start of this book, I said that the unique thing about running is that it offers seemingly limitless options: goals, distances, times, etc. All these options are worthy if they spark your passion.

I'm too old, or I came to the sport too late.

Maybe you believe you're too old to race, or if you've been racing since you were young, you see little point in continuing because all your best races are behind you. Maybe you'll need to adjust some of your expectations as the years march on, but that does not mean you can't accomplish things that will amaze yourself. There's always a new challenge yet to be explored.

Perhaps you came to the sport late and aren't entirely comfortable jumping into the fray, with the crowds and logistic hassles. Running is simple. Racing can add an element of fuss and bother that many aren't comfortable with. Or maybe you've never seen yourself as an athlete and think that only real athletes should race. In that case, test the waters a bit with a smaller race. See how it goes. See if you like it.

I don't know where to start.

While getting started with running seems like it should be easy and straightforward, when it comes to the shoes hitting the asphalt or the dirt, it turns out it may not be so easy. New runners often don't know where to start, how to start, or what to do first.

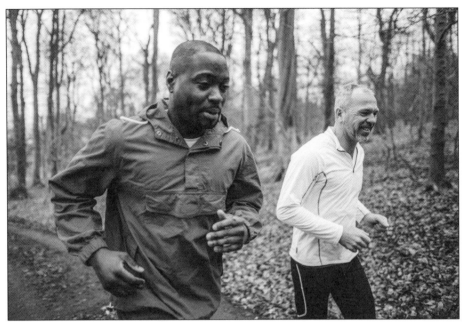

A great place to start is a local fun running group. In many areas, you can find weekly running groups at local running stores. Gyms also offer couch-to-5K sessions where you sign up with a group of people all working toward a 5K goal. These are led by coaches who will guide you on how to start, stay healthy, and get stronger. Local running groups, whether free community groups or coached running groups, also present the opportunity to connect with other runners and learn how to progress in running. I know many runners near me who have been running together as a group for years, sometimes traveling to the same races, but more importantly, providing accountability, encouragement, and education. If you enjoy this type of social interaction, this is a great option for you.

But perhaps you prefer to run solo most of the time, or maybe your schedule is complicated, so trying to get to a group run is difficult. In this case, you can do some research on your own or possibly hire a coach to guide you. There is a lot of running advice out there—books, YouTube videos, online training sites, Facebook, Instagram, Snapchat, influencers, running groups of all varieties, discussion boards, free training plans, blogs, podcasts, etc. Some of the advice is good, and some is not so good. The challenge is sifting through it all, separating the wheat from the chaff, and deciding what will work best for you.

The self-coached, newer runner (or even an experienced runner who has high aspirations or is taking on a new challenge) who doesn't have any experience with running must have a pretty insatiable appetite for and curiosity about the ever-changing information out there concerning training, nutrition, recovery, biomechanics, and injury rehab. That's why you're reading this book. But if you're thinking about getting help from a coach, whether in a group setting or individually, understand that coaches are not just for elite runners or those with audacious goals. They're for anyone who wants to learn, feel better, get stronger, and stay healthy.

I don't know how to set goals.

There are two main reasons that setting goals is important: (1) Goals provide focus, and (2) goals are motivating. But while it seems like it should be easy to set goals, that's not always the case. There are so many options, and it's hard to know if you're setting realistic goals.

As I've emphasized many times, the great thing about running is that there aren't really any rules on what qualifies as a goal. But like being presented with a 100-page menu at a restaurant, having so many choices can be paralyzing. Add to that the influence of social media and always seeing what others are doing, and it can leave you in a muddle. What do you want? What makes you excited (and maybe a little scared) when you think about it?

Here's the thing: You do not have to choose one thing to the exclusion of all other things. You can try out different goals. See if they fit or not, and then make subsequent choices from there. You also do not have to do everything now. Remember the annual plans and short-, medium-, and long-term goals discussed earlier. You may decide to do something that you later discover doesn't really inspire you, or maybe you enjoy it and find it rewarding for a time but then start thinking of other goals.

Think about what goals are reasonable given where you are right now. This is important because you don't want to set yourself up for a frustrating effort. If you started running this year and just ran your first 5K, does it make sense to set a goal for a marathon in six months? Maybe not. Maybe you'd benefit from spending more time building your aerobic base, increasing your speed, and learning about racing—a lot can happen during a race, and learning about the things that might pop up is as important as your training.

When you're just starting out, think about manageable, incremental goals, ones that push you a bit and also excite you. Goal that are measurable, achievable, and ambitious motivate you to keep getting out there and doing the work.

If you've been running for some time, then you have some experience with this—but that experience could be positive or negative. You need to set goals based on your history and your desire and ability to train, but not as a test of yourself against your younger self. Your younger self certainly matters here (see the section on age grading in chapter 2), but you are more than your younger self now. That is still part of you, but now your development is about where you are today, next month, next year, and five years from now.

I'm slow and afraid of coming in last.

The popular saying goes, "If you're out there, you're ahead of the person sitting on the couch." That by itself is an accomplishment. Another popular saying is, "A four-minute mile and an 18-minute (or any number) mile are both still a mile." I don't know too many runners who haven't feared they would come in last, but really—what does it matter?

A couple years ago, I ran the Ice Age Trail 50 in Wisconsin. This race has a long history and a loyal following and, with that, a fairly large field of capable runners. Now, I've run a lot of races. Some I've won, and most I have not, but I usually do okay. I've qualified for the Boston Marathon, New York City Marathon, and Chicago Marathon, all of which I've run several times. But on this unseasonably hot day in May, I was having a very hard day. The last couple miles, I wasn't sure I would get to the finish before the 12-hour cutoff, meaning an automatic DNF (did not finish) after 50 miles of agonizing effort—including a couple falls, one of which resulted in some dislocated ribs. The last half mile was grueling as I pushed with everything I had left, knowing that these 50 miles had now come down to mere seconds on the clock. I just wanted to stop. "What's the point?" I asked myself, but I kept pushing with all I had. I decided that either way, I would finish, even if I did not get an official finish. As I approached the finishing chute, the crowd was screaming furiously. I crossed the mat at 11:58:31 to the cheers of all those strangers and friends who had witnessed and appreciated what it looks like to give it your all even when things aren't going well.

The fact is, whether you're first or last, everyone runs the same run. You're there with your own goals, your own advantages and disadvantages, and you've been handed a day and a challenge to meet on your own terms.

It costs too much money and time.

This is certainly a barrier to entry when it comes to racing, but there are lots of options out there. Most race organizations offer free race entries for those who volunteer. Because most races rely heavily on volunteers, these opportunities are often easy to find, and volunteering is fun and rewarding. In fact, I believe that all runners who race should volunteer and give back to the community because when you run races, you depend on volunteers; without them, you wouldn't have all those wonderful races. There are also some free or inexpensive races out there. And for some runners, setting a budget for entry fees helps. Choose the races you really want and focus your effort and funds there.

I don't like crowds.
Small races, rural races without large spectator crowds, and trail races all generally have smaller crowds. Since the running boom of the 1970s, races have proliferated around the country and the world. The number of races on any given weekend, pretty much year-round and in all communities, offers so many options. Whether it's a local 5K charity race to support a worthy cause or a marathon through the countryside, you can find many races where you will be blissfully running alone to the sound of nature and your own thoughts.

Some of the reasons discussed here, I've mentioned or alluded to earlier as reasons to push past the challenges, fears, and doubts—the little voices in your head saying you can't do it or aren't good enough or are too old. It's important to recognize that those are fabrications and nothing more. So why race, or why set any specific goal? There are lots of very good reasons:

- Bring new motivation to your running
- See new places
- Challenge yourself
- Be part of a community
- Make or see friends
- Help charitable organizations and causes

For many runners of all ages, racing provides some motivation to get out there and run.

Racing also brings the running community together. I want to note that racing isn't a static thing. The value of racing can change over time. I raced a lot in my 20s and had very high expectations. But over time, those expectations undermined my enjoyment and my reason for racing. In my 40s, I jumped back into racing for very different reasons: to experience some iconic races in special places and to compete against myself, whatever that might mean on that day—perhaps to overcome a fear, to feel strong and competent, or even to run a fast (for me) time.

Selecting Your Race

Probably the most important question to ask yourself when it comes to selecting races is this: What do you want to do? When you're thinking about races, notice what makes you excited and maybe even a little nervous. Maybe you want to stay local, run for a good cause, see a new place, or try a different distance—but identifying what matters to you is the most important step in this process.

Then think about where you are now and where you want to be in three months, six months, 12 months, next year, and the year after that. Plan based on where you are now and where you want to be in the future.

Find the right challenge for you. What do I mean by "right"? I mean something that matters to you and presents a reasonable yet ambitious challenge. Something that makes you giddy and a bit terrified at the same time. Something that makes you smile at the very thought of it.

Discover What Excites You

I think this issue is not often addressed. It's not always easy figuring out what you want to do, even when it comes to running, something seemingly pure and simple. It seems straightforward, but it's not. Thanks to the internet and social media, the options are tantalizing and many, and the social pressure is not so easily dismissed. The fear of missing out (FOMO) is real.

The internet lets you easily search for races around the globe, and social media allows you to see all the cool things others are doing. There are clubs for runners who want to run in all 50 states—it could be a half-marathon, marathon, or any race. There's the World Marathon Majors, which currently includes Chicago, New York, Boston, London, Berlin, and Tokyo. There are clubs for people who want to rack up sub-three-hour or sub-four-hour marathons and clubs for sub-30-minute 5K runners. Whatever your heart desires, there's probably a club for it. But variety brings its own challenges in terms of listening to what really matters to you.

Here's a personal story: In 2016, I ran my third New York City Marathon (NYCM). The NYCM is very special to me because going to New York with my father to watch the marathon as a high school runner made a deep impression on me. I got back into racing at the age of 45 partially because I wanted to run New York. After several years of trying to get in via the lottery and failing, I decided to focus on trying to qualify. The times to qualify for automatic entry are faster than Boston qualifying times. I set up my training and racing to hopefully get me there. I succeeded in the fall of 2011 and was registered for 2012. About five days before the race, Hurricane Sandy hit the New York and New Jersey areas and caused massive destruction. The marathon was canceled, and so was my dream—or so I thought. After that experience, I decided I was done with NYCM.

But I wasn't. I qualified again in 2013, and at the last minute, I registered for the race. The 2013 NYCM was a blur. This was a race I had aspired to do for several decades. This was the race I had first thought about when the doctors told me at the age of 44 that I would never run again. And the crazy thing is that I cannot remember much of it. But it was part of a lifelong journey. This is what I wrote that night after the race:

November 3, 2013, 3:52 p.m.

I walk from Central Park, hop stiff-legged down the subway stairs, step onto the C line downtown to 34th Street, poke my head out from underground into the low fall light cut sharply by towering buildings, and make my way a couple blocks to Penn Station. I don't really want to leave. I want this to last. But I am tired and sticky with Gatorade.

The train pulls out from Penn Station, moving through the darkness deep beneath the Hudson River. All I can see in the window is my own reflection. My iPod seals me in my own little world, surrounded by people and their lives. I cannot talk to anyone right now. I need to be by myself. The train emerges from underground into the yellow late-afternoon autumn light and through the marshlands. Cattails and tall yellow-brown grasses gently bend in the breeze. Hawks glide by on invisible waves. I am struck to tears by the beauty of this place, a place I have always seen as ugly, ruined, defiled, sad. The sky is a hazy autumn blue. The whole world is soft and gentle around the edges. And after more than 30 years of rejecting the very idea of this place as part of me, I find myself overwhelmed by a thankfulness that hits me as a sudden shock. I have spent so much time pretending this is not me, and yet it is me. This place, the environment, the people—I owe them all gratitude for this day.

When Socrates is sentenced to death by his fellow Athenians and sent to jail to await his hemlock, he is given ample opportunity to leave. The jailer leaves the doors unlocked and open. Freedom is one step away. His students beg him to leave and save himself. They cry at his side, pleading with him to leave. He will not. He sees himself as who he is because of Athens, its people, its culture—this time and this place is what made him what he is. He would not be the person he is without these people, this place, this time. And so, he accepts, though he does not agree with, the judgment and punishment handed down by those who made him who he is. And the jailer brings him his hemlock, and he drinks it and dies, with his students sobbing at his bedside. And Socrates dies, as he believes he must, to remain Socrates. Anything else entails a sacrifice of his very self.

What makes us what we are—who we are?

Today will not sink in to my brain. Try as I may, it will not happen. My brain pushes it away. While running, I say to myself, "My god, you're here. This is it!" My brain says, "Yeah, so what?" But in my skin, my throat, my heart, my soul, I am lost in it—the blur of being in it. Sometimes we look forward to something but fail to be there, truly there, when it happens. How to be there? The brain just can't grasp it. It's too much, and it's really nothing. It is nothing at all. Running through the streets of New York City is pretty unspectacular. Anyone can do this any day of the year. I am simply running down a city street.

What an experience is for anyone is dependent on the person and the experience. It is nothing but that.

For me, this is even more than I know, than I knew when I began all this, and I feel that sink in as I sit on this train passing the refineries, the long-ago-shuttered factories, the razor-wire fences, the men smoking cigarettes, laughing and shooting baskets. The small grocery shops, the old woman pushing a shopping cart along the cracked-to-bits sidewalks. The windowless lounge, a neon martini glass flickering against the red brick wall. After last year, 2012, when the NYC Marathon was canceled at the last minute due to Hurricane Sandy, a first in the history of this much esteemed marathon, and the ensuing NYCM fiasco that followed, I washed my hands of all this. Then I thought again.

Thirty-five years after taking this same train line into NYC with my father to witness Grete Waitz's first victory in New York, I am heading home having done what I told myself I would do on that day. I am going back to the house I went back to then. Most of this area, on the surface, is unchanged from the '70s, when all these factories began shutting down. Nothing has really changed. Everything always changes. What remains through the passing of time is us. We remain.

Aristotle asks us to consider this: Take a ship. Replace every bit of the ship with new pieces—every board, every nail, every itty-bitty piece. Is it now the same ship it was? Good question. There is not a single cell in my body that is the same as any cell in my body 35 years ago. In this sense, we all have become many different people over the years. And yet, I am the same person, and today I came to an important realization: This place I rejected with such vehemence, I now embrace as the very core of who I have become—what makes life and a self really matter. I may not like it all, but it is me, good or bad, and I need to accept that. This place made me who I am, as did running, and it made me the runner I was and am and will be and the person I was and am and will be. And I guess I'm usually okay with all that.

My father had no idea what he did for me back in 1978. But I now know at least a piece of it.

My father is gone now. But at this moment, he is with me, sitting beside me, as he was 35 years ago on this very day, going home with me, having given me the chance—planting a seed that burst open, took root, and grew—to do something that really matters to me. And once again, I am changed by the experience.

This race had and has so much meaning for me, and it directed many of my actions for several years. The next year, I ran it again, this time running with a friend and really taking it all in. I registered again for 2016, but as the race approached, I started feeling like I wasn't sure why I was running it. Did I just feel I needed to run it every time I could? Partially, I wanted to be a 10-year NYCM runner, but that really wasn't very compelling for me. I realized going in that I had done what I had set out to do there, and now I was kind of forcing the issue. I remember thinking I would not have run that year had I not already paid the (substantial) entry fee.

At that moment, I realized I had lost my way, my why (more on that later), and the excitement that comes with it. After 2016, I said that I might run NYCM again, but only for a very special reason. And yet, every year as I see friends getting ready to run it, there is this little pang of desire. It's still there under the surface, and maybe it will roar again.

There's a lot out there vying for your attention: friends asking you to run a race with them, cool races in cool places, events that seem to be on everyone's bucket list. The internet, social media, and even local running groups can provide inspiration and exciting options, or they may distract you from the things you find most compelling.

Social media brought me literally thousands of new running friends from all over the world—some of whom I've met over the years and others I hope to meet. I've heard the tales of others' heroic feats, and to some extent, this exposure broadens my own horizons. My running world is so much bigger now than it was 20 years ago. I see what others who are not so different from me are able to do. The influence of social media on running and on how you direct your individual running goals can be beneficial or detrimental.

Choose Your Challenge

You must always be mindful of your own goals, wants, desires, and needs. Your achievements are your achievements. My achievements are my achievements. My greatest competitor is myself. In some cases, seeing what others are doing can undermine your feelings about your own achievements. The claim that comparison is the thief of joy is all the truer in the age of instant connection.

Recently, there was a thread on a Facebook running group page about people who run races but don't actually *race* them—or at least claim not to race them but rather use these races as workouts. There are some runners who don't understand this idea of running a race while not always *racing* it—as in, not giving it your best possible effort. Some judge others on how they choose to run a race, implying that it's simply inappropriate.

The same applies to comments about running a race even if you are better off not starting. The claim that a DNF is always better than a DNS (did not start) is not a helpful view. Sometimes, it's better to just not start, especially if you are dealing with an injury or illness.

I enjoy running races as part of my training for goal races. I often run shorter races while training for a marathon or ultra. It's helpful for me for several reasons: First, I tend to push myself harder when I'm racing, even if I'm not racing all out. It's easier to get a good tempo run, lactate-threshold run, or marathon-pace run done this way. Second, it keeps me in racing mode, so to speak, where I'm pressed to keep pushing to the end even when I'm feeling tired. Out on a training run, I'm much more likely to give in when the going gets tough. Third, it allows me to test my fueling and pacing plan. Finally, as a fairly solitary runner with a complicated schedule that makes it difficult for me to run with others, I like being around other runners, and racing is an opportunity to be more social. I like the running community and look forward to these training races.

I find this to be a good way to get my racing fix without racing myself into an injury, all the while keeping my eye on the prize: the goal race that is most important to me. But sometimes, I have a hard time not pushing as hard as I can because that's the common expectation. And that's also when training discipline matters. You'll have to learn that discipline because you'll need it for your race.

With all that said, the main takeaway here is to always listen to your voice first. Maybe your running group is planning to run a race together that you just aren't excited about, or maybe the race doesn't excite you but running with your friends does, or maybe both sound like fun. Maybe there's a race you've heard about that sounds really intriguing. Add it to your list. See how it will fit into your life and training.

Choose a Race That Fits Your Life

Running should not be just another chore you add to your to-do list. If running becomes another obligation you *must* do, then you probably won't keep doing it. Running is something you *get* to do. If you find yourself saying, "I *have* to do my run," then you need to look at how your running fits in with the rest of your life and why you are really doing it.

Do you like to train in the heat? Do you like to train in the cold? Are there schedule or life demands at certain times of the year that make training more difficult—or easier? Will you have the time you need to prepare for the race you choose? Will you need to make adjustments, and are you willing to do so?

For many runners 50 and over, there may be fewer family demands because children are likely older and sometimes able to look after themselves—but if you have teenagers, shuttling them around can still be fairly demanding. Or perhaps you help with grandchildren or an older family member. Considering these demands, there may be times of the year when it's easier to train.

As an example, depending on work demands, some parents of older kids do better training during the school year, when schedules are more predictable. During the summer, finding time for training can be more challenging with vacations and changing schedules for older kids or grandkids. Or maybe you'd just rather do other things during the summer, so summer training would be your down season.

Maybe you have a job with seasonal demands that change. Lots of jobs have high and low seasons, and learning which times of the year suit serious training is important. If running becomes just another stressor, it's going to be unpleasant, and you won't stick with it. This is most often learned the hard way when you push yourself through a training cycle and hate the whole process. It doesn't need to be that way.

Perhaps you hate running in the heat, so summer running is just not enjoyable. Or you hate running in the cold and snow and ice, so winter is out. Again, this is very individual, and part of the decision process is learning what works best for you.

You may be willing to make some sacrifices for a race you really want to do, even if it doesn't come at the optimal time. Knowing what you're getting yourself into, however, is important. Understanding that it won't be easy but that you are committed to a goal will get you out there when you might otherwise give up.

Once you identify the best times of the year to train, then you have to determine whether you have sufficient time to prepare based on where you are now. This is one very good reason to think about goals over a period of a year or more. Maybe you want to run a marathon in four months, but do you have time to prepare for that based on your running now? Should you instead think about a half-marathon and then plan for a marathon later?

It's okay to take time to decide what your goals are and what works best for your life as a whole. Many simply assume these things are easy, straightforward decisions, but I've seen many runners experience times where they feel adrift and unsure about what to do next. They often feel like it should be obvious, but sometimes things that appear simple are not. I've seen runners get caught up in a groupthink—they start going along with what others are doing, only to realize somewhere along the line that they really aren't into what they're doing. Lots of people flippantly say, "Just run." But if you just run, you may find yourself frustrated, dealing with injuries, stagnating progress, and flagging motivation. It's okay to sit back for a time and think about your options and what you want to do. It may not come to you instantly, and that's okay. There are so many paths you can take, and sometimes variety leads to indecision as you ponder all the options.

It's easy to choose a meal when there are only a few items on the menu. When you are presented with dozens of tantalizing options, trying to pick just one is difficult—but you can always try one now and then come back and try another. Approaching running with the big picture in mind allows you to focus on one thing and dream about all the others yet to come. Whether you are in your 50s, 60s, 70s, or beyond, I strongly believe that pursuing your goals and having more lined up keeps you young and motivated to go after your dreams.

Chapter 13

Designing Your Race-Day Strategy

You've spent weeks and months training for this day, but now you need a race-day plan. This plan will include things like specific goals for the race, prerace warm-up and nutrition, race pacing and nutrition, postrace recovery, and postrace analysis. Planning for your race day should begin a couple weeks out from your goal race and should be fine-tuned a couple days before.

Don't forget to include a celebration—for getting here, for accepting a challenge that pushed you out of your comfort zone, and for training on the days you didn't want to. Getting to the starting line is an accomplishment in itself, and getting to the finish is the celebration.

Setting Race-Day Goals

As I have discussed in earlier chapters, setting goals can and should be done during training. However, they must be reexamined and adjusted before the race, looking at where your training has taken you, how you've responded, how you're feeling going into the race, and what is reasonable to aim for based on the training block you have completed. You may have responded so well to your training—hitting your workouts and paces better than expected—that you can adjust your goal to be more ambitious. Or perhaps life demands or sickness interfered with your training in ways you could not foresee when you began. As the race gets closer, you also need to consider weather conditions and other contributing factors such as any recent illness, injury, or life stressors. All may require an adjustment of expectations either up or down.

Goals can be tweaked even during the race if you have been thoughtful about your goals. Things can happen during races, and the longer the race, the more likely that becomes. Part of training—along with accrued experience and adding in training races when appropriate—is learning how to be adaptable. Sometimes you need to adjust in the moment.

Here's an example: One year that I ran the NYCM, I prepared well, with all my gear and fuel ready and my plan in place. The start was chilly, so I added a pair of arm sleeves for a little warmth for the opening miles. My intention was to toss the arm sleeves once the temperature rose. I tend to prefer running with as little stuff as possible, so I usually tuck my gels into the small pockets in my shorts, but this time I tucked them under my arm sleeves. At about the 5K mark, I had warmed up enough, so I peeled off the sleeves and tossed them (this is common in marathons; the race often allows this and collects the clothing for donation). A few miles down the road, when it came time for me to take a gel, it suddenly hit me that I had tossed the gels with the sleeves. My fueling plan had flown off with my sleeves, and I suddenly had to replan on the run. Since the NYCM didn't have a gel station until mile 19 that year, I had to rely on the course Gatorade. This was not optimal since I had not trained with Gatorade and it's not my preference, but I didn't have other options. I remember running behind other runners, spying gel packets tucked into their hydration belts and feeling envious and a little stupid. But I didn't let my error derail the race. I had done the important work of knowing what fuel would be offered on the course and when it would be offered. If I had waited, hoping for gels at the water stations, I probably would have run out of energy before getting there. Things happen that you can't anticipate, and even the best plan can fall apart. Learning to be flexible and being willing to problem-solve are underrated but important skills in running.

Going into your race, you need to have several goals. I recommend setting three goals:

- *A goal:* Your A goal is what you'd like to do on a perfect day, where you feel fantastic and able to reach the highest level of your ability.
- *B goal:* Your B goal is what is reasonable but still demanding.
- *C goal:* Your C goal is what you will walk away satisfied with even if your day does not go as planned.

Having different goals allows you to adjust based on the day you're handed. Humans are not machines, and just like in training, there are days you feel like you're flying and days you are dragging, and sometimes the cause is not clear. In pursuing any goal, you need to have a range of expectations that still allow for satisfaction and growth.

Prerace and Race Nutrition

The general rule in racing is to never change anything on race day. If you've been doing things that work in training, try to keep those consistent on race day. If you have a prerun breakfast that works for you in training, eat that before your race and allow the same amount of time to digest it as you would allow in training. Use the fuel and hourly calorie count you've been using during training.

Expect that you may have some prerace jitters, which can cause an unsettled stomach for some, but not eating is not a wise choice. Instead, allow enough time to slowly eat your prerace food.

I recommend taking in some quick-to-digest calories about 15 minutes before the start of the race, just to top off the tank. This can be a gel, some chews with water, or some liquid fuel. As with everything, this should be tested in training, especially before runs that require a comparable effort level as your race—so speed sessions or tempo runs are ideal for testing your gut tolerance. For novices with little speed and tempo work, try this before a few of your longer runs.

In terms of nutrition during the race, for shorter races such as a 5K or 10K, going in well-fueled is recommended, and taking in some calories on the run can help you maintain energy. Since you will be running harder for shorter races, be careful to eat and drink things that are easy to digest. Gels, chews, and liquids are best for short, intense races. For longer races such as half-marathons and longer, aim for somewhere between 150 and 300 calories an hour. Different runners will be able to tolerate different amounts of calories, and this should be tested in training. Once you find the right number for you, stick with that during the race.

How you manage nutrition during the race will depend on several factors:

- Will you use the fuel options offered on the course? If so, train with the products offered at your race and make sure they work for you.
- If you are using course fuel options, how far apart are the fuel and aid stations? Will that be enough for you, or will you need to carry some hydration and fuel with you?
- Are you bringing your own fuel or nutrition? If so, have a plan for what you will need.
- Do you plan to use a hydration pack or belt, or do you prefer a handheld bottle?
- Will you refill your bottle during the race?

Race-Day Routines

Some runners have race-day routines that help calm the nerves. If you have a set way of getting ready, it becomes almost like a ritual, and you will be less likely to forget something. Rituals and routines take time to develop, but once you establish them, you have a habitual checklist of sorts. It can be something as simple as eating a specific breakfast, listening to a song, visualizing yourself running strong, going for a short warm-up run, or wearing certain clothes—whatever brings comfort and calm into the routine.

As an example, years ago, my daughter made me a bracelet. She must have been three or four at the time, and it was around Halloween, so it has Halloween colors. Halloween is her favorite time of year, so that bracelet had special meaning for me. It was just a simple black-

and-orange cord, but I wore it every day and for every race. I wore that bracelet for years, until it became threadbare, and then I wore it only for important races. It now sits in a secure box, protected and only taken out for special races. When I'm getting ready for a race, I take that cord from its box and put it on. This is part of my prerace ritual. As I'm getting ready, it helps ground and calm me. That cord around my wrist reminds me what really matters to me when things get hard. When I ran my first 100-miler, the last seven miles required everything I had in me and more. That last seven miles seemed almost impossible at the time. What got me through those miles was looking at that cord wrapped around my wrist and thinking of my young daughter, still warm in bed at home, and about telling her that I had done it. Almost 10 years later, I wore it for what would end up being my fastest 100-miler. As with that first one, when things got hard, I looked at that cord around my wrist and was reminded about what really mattered. My daughter is now 15 years old, but still the thought of her reminds me of what's important and of the people who matter and support me. Sometimes those simple reminders keep you grounded and focused when you most need it.

Similarly, some runners use mantras—meaningful sayings that can bring you back to focus at different times. Mantras can become cues for motivation when you're going through a tough patch, help you check in on your running form, and return you to focusing on the goal instead of allowing your mind to wander off to negative thoughts about how hard it feels or if you can do what you want to do. I can't tell you how many times I've been in the opening miles of a race and thought, "Why do I do this to myself?" It's natural when you're uncomfortable to forget the important things you care about. Here are some common mantras:

   I can do hard things.
   Light and fast.
   I get to do this.
   Pain is temporary. Quitting is forever.
   Breathe.
   I will finish.
   I am strong.
   I trained for this.
   Be fierce.
   Embrace the suck.
   Right, left, repeat.
   I want that medal.

A mantra can be anything that brings you back to why you signed up and set off on this journey in the first place. Your mind likes to protect you from stress, so sometimes it wants to shut the whole thing down before you really want to give up.

Warming Up

For any race shorter than a marathon, a good running warm-up is recommended to warm up your muscles, tendons, and ligaments, get your metabolism moving, increase your heart rate and the blood flow to your muscles, and bring in more oxygen. As I mentioned previously, the shorter the race, the longer the warm-up. The harder you're going to be running from the start, the more you need that warm-up. For a 5K, depending on your goals and your mileage in training, a warm-up could be anywhere from one to three miles at an aerobic pace (based on the training you have been doing), ending with several fast strides (three or four 10-second strides). If you are a novice racer, an easy mile ending with three or four 10-second strides is good. For a seasoned racer, three miles of easy running with four or five 10- to 20-second strides is good. For a 10K, a warm-up could be anywhere from one to two miles plus the strides from the 5K warm-up. For half-marathons, I recommend 5 to 10 minutes of easy running plus four or five strides of 10 to 20 seconds each.

For marathons and longer distances, doing some dynamic warm-ups (see chapter 8 for suggestions) for three to five minutes gets your blood moving and your muscles warmed up before the start. Then, because marathon pace is a lower intensity, using the first mile or so to get up to pace generally works well. For marathons, some dynamic stretches will be adequate to increase your heart rate and blood flow.

Race Pacing

Pacing is a skill that must be learned like any other skill. Many runners think they will naturally know what pace to run, but learning consistent pacing should be part of your training. Assuming you've done this, getting ready for a race involves deciding on a pacing plan based on your training and then sticking to that plan. This means you must trust and believe in your plan.

Before I get into the specifics of race pacing, let me explain some terminology and approaches to racing:

- *Negative splits:* Run the second half (later miles) of the race faster than the first half (early miles).

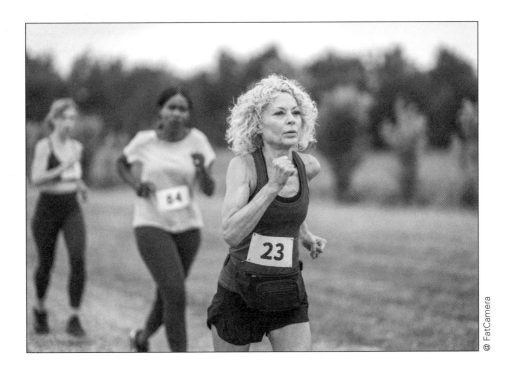

- *Positive splits:* Run faster for the first half (opening miles) and slower for the second half (later miles).
- *Even splits:* Run the first half and the second half at the same pace.

There's lots of discussion on which of the above approaches is better. But based on research and statistics, most runners see better results aiming for negative splits. This applies most often to half-marathons and marathons. There's a bit more variability with races shorter than a half-marathon, and most runners do not run negative splits in ultras—though for a flat 50K, you can approach it similar to a road marathon.

5K Through Half-Marathon Pacing

For these races, you have hopefully done some runs during training that give you an idea of what you are capable of running. These include 800- to 1,500-meter intervals, repeats, and shorter tempo runs. These runs are paced based on your goals. If you can complete those runs at the designated paces, you should be on target for your goal race pace. Both 5Ks and 10Ks are run at a fairly hard effort from the start. Based on the key workouts you do in training, such as intervals and repeats, you will have an idea of what you can run for your race. You should aim for your goal race pace plus or minus 10 seconds per mile.

Terrain will also come into play. If your race has hills, you will run a bit slower uphill and faster downhill. For a flat race, starting out just a little slower than your aimed pace and then pressing harder with each mile tends to result in the best outcome. Taking off at a sprint at the beginning of your race will likely leave you slowing down for the rest of the race rather than speeding up; the seconds you bank at the beginning of the race are usually lost many times over later in the race.

Marathon Pacing

Picture this scenario: You are standing on the starting line, blood rushing through your veins, legs jumpy with anticipation, bouncing foot to foot—champing at the bit—and the gun fires. You cross the mats, press the start button on your GPS watch, and take off with the flow of runners. What could be more natural? You're running with energy and speed—light on your feet. Your breath and feet and legs and heart are all there in the moment. You feel so good.

And then you take a quick glance at your wrist. Your target pace is 8:15, but the watch screen indicates you are at about 7:50. "Sweet," you think. "I'm ahead of pace, and I feel great. I feel so flipping great! This is my day. I am going to crush that PR." And so it goes for the first six miles, at which point you begin to wonder if perhaps you pushed it a bit too fast. So you pull back on the reins and settle into your projected 8:15 pace. That feels okay for another 10 miles, but then you notice your pace begins to drop a bit. You're struggling to stay on target, and your legs are beginning to feel a little heavy. You try harder, but your legs just don't respond. Now you're at 8:40 and struggling to maintain that. You start to feel a little panicky. At mile 21, your pace drops to 9:10, then 9:20 . . . You walk-run your way to the finish. You feel like you're crawling and cannot will your legs to move any faster. How can something that began so gloriously end in ignominious defeat?

For shorter distances, you may get away with making some pacing errors, but the marathon distance is unforgiving. Generally, your optimal marathon pace is very close to, but slightly slower than, your lactate-threshold (LT) pace. Why? There are two reasons, really (I discussed this earlier, but it's crucial to remind yourself of it during the race):

1. Once you drop down to a pace just a bit faster than your LT pace, certain physiological things begin happening. In your muscles, acid concentration increases. This interferes with energy production and muscle contraction. Stay just above (run a bit slower than) your LT, and that lactate is used to produce more ATP, the energy source you need to keep your muscles

contracting. Lactate is a fuel, but when there's too much produced at once, then it cannot be taken up fast enough and accumulates in your muscles. This is the big problem. Lactate is not the enemy; too much lactate produced too fast is the enemy. That accumulating lactate creates an acidic environment that physically damages your muscles and interferes with the process of muscle contraction.

2. When you stay just above your LT, you can use both fat and glycogen for energy production. Go under your LT, and you predominantly rely on glycogen, which is a very limited fuel source. If you can stay in the zone where both fat and glycogen are used, sparing the limited glycogen for as long as possible, then you are less likely to hit a wall at mile 17, 20, or 22. Contrary to popular opinion, hitting a wall during a marathon is not necessary—it tells you that you are making a pacing mistake, a fueling mistake, or both.

So, let's return to the previous scenario. Let's say you run just five seconds per mile faster than your LT for the first six miles of the marathon. What happens then? The environment in your muscles is now acidic, and that shuts down the enzymes needed for ATP production. You feel heavy and tight. And now you must work harder to maintain the pace that would have felt doable had you not begun this whole metabolic domino process. You have also burned through precious glycogen at a higher rate than you needed to, so you'll run out of it earlier in the race. The result is that the seconds you banked during the early stages of the race will be lost many times over during the later stages of the race.

Training, of course, should aim to lower the pace at which you can run before hitting your LT—that is, you should be training to improve your LT pace—and your race pace should be determined with that in mind. But it is crucial that you stay above that place where bad things begin to happen. The problem is that you will not feel the deleterious effects until after it is too late. Once the damage is done, there's no way to quickly undo it. It takes time that you just don't have during the race.

Most runners have experienced the consequences of going out too fast, and yet they continue to do it. It takes discipline and understanding to do the right thing, especially when everyone around you is doing the wrong thing by going out too fast. But I guarantee that if you heed this warning, you will pass all those suffering through the later stages of their race—and best of all, you will feel stronger and more capable than you ever have before.

Ultramarathon Pacing

An ultramarathon is, by definition, any distance longer than a marathon; most ultras range between 50 kilometers and 100 miles. The pacing plan for an ultra race (and this can apply to any distance trail race as well) depends on the distance and the demands of that specific course. Unlike a road race, which may contain some demanding hills, trail races (the usual terrain for ultra races) may also involve technical running terrain: rocks, roots, slickrock, and very steep terrain. With ultras and trail races, running based on perceived effort rather than a preset pace plan is often the best tactic. Pacing based on perceived effort and the specific demands of the race you're running must be part of your training.

How you pace a 50K and a 100-miler will vary greatly. While all ultras tend to be lumped into the same category, they are very different beasts depending on distance and course-specific demands. There is no one approach for all ultra-distance runs. For that reason, I like to distinguish between shorter and longer ultras: The shorter range from 50K to 50 miles, and the longer range from 50 miles to 100 miles (or up to about 125 miles). Races well beyond 100 miles require additional considerations.

With any ultra, you want to pay attention to the following:

- *Vertical gain:* Make sure you know how many feet your goal race will climb and descend. The term *gain* usually refers to the number of vertical feet for only the ascents. *Elevation change*, or similar terms, often covers both ascent and descent. It's important to know both the gain and loss because you need to train for both.
- *Technical demands:* What terrain does your race include? Is it a rail-trail course with few technical obstacles? Is it a smooth single-track trail? Does it include highly technical terrain? Is it a mix of more and less runnable terrain?
- *Typical weather conditions:* Heat, rain, snow, and wind all figure into how you approach pacing. A normally mellow single-track dirt trail can turn into a slippery, muddy mess in rain. Heat and humidity always require adjustments.

50K to 50 Miles Pacing

Running a 50K with 1,000 feet of vertical gain and running a 50K with 9,000 feet of gain require very different approaches to pacing. For a nontechnical, relatively flat 50K, depending on your training, your pace can be similar to what you would run for a marathon. Running a

50K with 9,000 feet of gain and added technical terrain calls for much different pacing.

Likewise, for flat 50-milers, you may find you're able to run a fair amount of it. But since 50 miles is likely quite a bit farther than you've run in training, you need to be very careful not to blow yourself up over the first half. While you may be able to run a flat 50K a little slower than LT pace, for a 50-miler you will likely be running closer to your comfortable aerobic pace while possibly adding in some walking breaks along the way. What's important for these long nontechnical runs is to keep your effort feeling very comfortable from the start. When paced well, these shorter nontechnical ultras can be run at a fairly even pace.

For runs involving lots of elevation gain and technical running, you need to set your pace based on effort. Long, steep climbs will involve fast hiking (or sometimes just putting one foot in front of the other) while taking full advantage of more runnable sections. Being able to change gears based on terrain is important. What I recommend in these cases is to run until it feels too hard and then walk until it feels too easy.

For most longer ultras, some fast hiking will be required. One of the ever-present myths in ultra running is that flat races are easy and those with a lot of climbing constitute hard races. On the face of it, this may have some truth, but too many runners fall prey to this idea and end up making bad pacing choices. Also, what makes something hard or easy depends on the effort applied. For example, it's very easy to run yourself into a bad situation in flat 100-milers. Unlike courses with a lot of ascents and descents, flatter courses don't offer natural hiking cues, so many runners don't take walk breaks early. In this case, perceived effort can sometimes get you in trouble. This is a time for setting up a run-walk plan with scheduled walk breaks added in before you feel they are needed. One example is to run for eight minutes, walk for two minutes, then repeat. When this starts feeling hard, adjust. I prefer a distance schedule rather than a time schedule: When you hear a mile indicator beep on your watch, walk one-tenth to two-tenths of a mile (0.2K to 0.4K), then run easy until the next mile beep. Repeat. These can be adjusted as needed.

Keep in mind that, particularly for runners over 50, course-specific technical skills such as fast hiking and quick, light downhill running require specific training to develop. For older runners, muscle strength and mobility decrease over time. Working to maintain both is crucial for feeling confident on difficult terrain. Adding strength and mobility work to your training, in addition to training on course-specific terrain, will help you maintain your ability to complete these races with confidence and a reduced risk of injury.

Running a race does not stop with training. Smart racing is just as crucial as the weeks and months of doing the work to hit your runs, recover well, and then taper. Planning for race logistics, fueling, pacing, and the course itself is just as important as your training. Add in unexpected events, weather, and life stresses, and you'll realize there are things you can control and things you cannot. Plan for the things you can control, and accept and learn how to deal with the things you can't control. Having your race plan in hand is part of controlling what you can control, and it will result in the best race experience. If you've done the training and the race planning, you have what it takes to succeed.

Chapter 14

Staying Focused and Avoiding Setbacks

Running is not easy. A common joke about running is that it's the punishment used in other sports, and unfortunately that's how many are introduced to it. Running is not easy physically, and it's not easy mentally. Staying consistent day after day, even on those days when you just don't want to, can feel like a grind at times. But running is also a time for mental recharge—a time with and by yourself, a time of deep and meaningful conversation with friends, or a time to sort through life challenges. Knowing why you're doing it is crucial. It can be a race goal. It can be a fitness goal. It can be a connection with yourself. It can be a meetup with friends. But running must hold some meaningful space in your life.

Whether you aim to run your first 5K or your first 100-miler or you just want to establish a regular running habit, understanding your *why* matters. Your why is what helps you get out the door when you don't want to go and keeps you moving when you want to stop. Recognizing your why is the first step to developing a habit that will allow you to achieve your goals. Having goals is great, but knowing they are goals that *matter to you* is even more important.

One of the challenges of finding or creating your why is tapping into your deepest desires. Sometimes it's hard to truly identify your desires in a world full of options. Sometimes there's just so much noise around you—other runners, social media, etc. It's hard to listen to your own internal voice.

> None of us will ever accomplish anything excellent or commanding except when he listens to this whisper which is heard by him alone.
>
> *Ralph Waldo Emerson*

But finding or creating your why is all about you and no one else. Today many runners bemoan FOMO (fear of missing out) about what others around them are doing, but your why needs to come from you. Your why is not a static thing; it will change as your personal experiences grow and change, but it is always grounded in your individual values and desires—what matters most to you and what you find most interesting, exciting, and motivating. But discovering, uncovering, creating, and knowing how to act on these desires and values are not always straightforward.

Understand Process Versus Outcome

While setting goals (the outcome) can keep you moving forward, if you are not enjoying the process of getting to those goals, you will likely not keep at it for long. You will also measure success or failure based on a very narrow result. This approach downplays the value found in the process.

This brings up the concept of ends and means. You can do something as a means to an end—aiming at the end alone—or you can do it as an end in itself. If you enjoy running, then the very act of running is something you seek to do regardless of some further goal. If you are only focused on the goal, then the means of getting there offers little value. If, however, you find value in both the process and the outcome, your experience is richer, and the outcome is more flexible. End goals are often black and white: You either succeed or fail. Process goals can be progressive, fluid, and adaptive.

So now, I want to talk about the process, which requires a level of faith for all runners who have dreams and goals and wishes and aspirations. Whatever your goals are, you take risks by investing in those dreams. But the acts of faith along the way, which take you down the path toward your goals, matter. I have seen runners devastated after failing to reach their end goal. They lament: all that training, all that time, all that effort—wasted. All for nothing.

Several years ago, I ran Boston 2 Big Sur, an event where you run the Boston Marathon on the East Coast and then, six days later (it's longer some years, but not the year I ran), run the Big Sur International Marathon on the West Coast—a coast-to-coast adventure. My goal was to race Boston hard and have fun at Big Sur. Meanwhile, I was using both as training for my first 100-mile race.

The weather in Boston that year was horrendous, with temperatures in the low 40s, torrential rain, and strong headwinds the entire race. I ran decently well, but not what I knew I could do on a better day. Six days later, still feeling a little disappointed about Boston, I decided to give Big Sur a decent effort, and that lasted for about 10 miles until accumulating fatigue finally reared its ugly head, along with gale-force headwinds that literally ripped race bibs off runners' bodies. I put my head down and pressed on, stopping occasionally to take in the breathtaking views that Big Sur is so famous for.

After the race, many friends reached out to congratulate me: "You must be so happy." I was happy, but I was also disappointed. Things had not gone as I'd hoped. Being dealt a bad weather day is always a risk you hope won't happen. But it does happen, and you need to deal with it and adjust your expectations. While I was disappointed, it never occurred to me to think that all my training was a waste of time.

Training is a tricky, trying business. Training for races means toughing it out through trying conditions—rain, cold, heat, or wind—and days when you're tired or have to make time because you don't have any. You invest a lot in your goals. This investment is the result of faith:

believing that it matters and that it will make a difference, even when there are no guarantees. Even when the whole plan can evaporate before your eyes due to weather, illness, or injury, you still go out there and try, day in and day out. You give it your all and hope for the best. So, as you approach a race or another goal, you may know what you are capable of, and you may have put in the work, but that's only part of the story. You also need to have a good day.

What else can you do? You can't control the uncontrollable. You can't really function thinking, "Well, maybe I'll skip this tempo run because the day of the race might suck anyway, so why even try?" Runners don't think that way. Runners are, by very nature, optimistic and hopeful. You would never go out, day after day, working hard when you'd rather not, pushing on through it all, if you didn't have faith that it mattered. But the fact remains that often you get handed a totally bad day. Maybe the weather is bad, or you just don't feel well. But does that mean all that time training, running, and thinking about goals was a waste of time? I don't think so. And hopefully, the next day, you wake up and start concocting plans for the next one.

There are always going to be some goals you reach and others you fall short of. That's the risk of trying, reaching, and dreaming. But it's the reaching that matters. It's the effort that matters—the life, the energy. You live in the pursuit of what is best in yourself. What's the real alternative? You can set your sights nice and safe and low and achieve them all, pat yourself on the back for achieving things that really didn't demand much of you, and never know what you could really do. Or you can go for the wildly outrageous, crazy, pie-in-the-sky goals that get your spine tingling. Ambitious goals are the key to improvement and progress.

> The future depends on what you do today.
>
> *Mahatma Gandhi*

When someone comes to me—worried about some uncontrollable something they may be facing for an upcoming race, bemoaning their bad luck in being dealt a bad day, afraid they might have a bad day come race day, concerned they'll fall short of their goal, or lamenting that their goals are too grand—and says, "I wasted all that time training," all I can say is, "That's the nature of the beast. It's what you do. A lot of times, it sucks. A lot of times, it may not suck, but it's not great either. And sometimes—not often, but sometimes—it all comes together at just the right time." And *that* is why you have faith and keep reaching for the things that matter to you.

All runners who pursue their aims must share this faith in the future while finding the present satisfying in itself. It makes you more alive

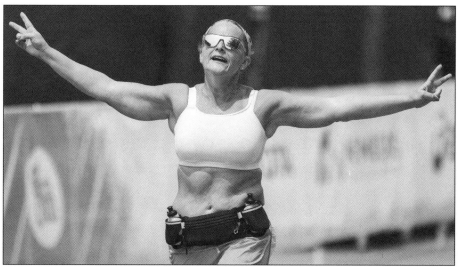

every day and keeps you moving forward, even when you feel like you're being pushed down by fickle luck, injury, illness, and even aging. Your actions, not your words, show what you really believe. And when you continue pursuing the things that matter to you, those actions show that you believe in what's possible. You have faith that it will happen, even when you have no assurance and no guarantee, even when the odds are against you and fate slaps you down. You get right back up on that horse and point yourself in the direction of that next big thing.

If all that matters is the end—the goal, and that goal is all-or-nothing—then you will likely feel that it's all been a waste if you don't reach that goal.

Believe in Yourself

Successful athletes—those who see themselves as successfully pursuing their goals, whatever those goals are—understand that attitude and outlook is a choice. Generally, those who maintain a positive attitude enjoy the process and find satisfaction in the outcome, whether that's reaching a desired goal, learning an important lesson, or both. They see competition as a personal journey, seeking mastery over perfection. They set goals based on their deepest desires and what really drives them and matters to them.

While you must do the physical training to reach your goals, going into the training and the race believing in yourself is also essential to a positive process and outcome. You must believe you can deal with the (often self-imposed) demands placed on you and handle the possible obstacles that may present themselves, some of which are completely unpredictable and novel. Part of this is also believing in your training and what your training indicates you are capable of doing and then trusting that and acting on it. At the end of a training cycle, you may have an idea of what you're able to run, but then you must be willing to take some risks and go after what you are confident you can do.

Practice Mental Imagery and Visualization

Successful athletes can use training and racing to mentally transport themselves to a place of strength and success. Seeing yourself running strong and feeling capable is important going into a race. As an example of this, I encourage you to do some of your more demanding training runs on terrain and at an effort level that will mimic your race-day experience. During the race, you can then mentally transport yourself to that physical place, that training run, where you felt strong and crushed the workout. You can also use a shorter workout to transport yourself to the end miles of your race, where you discover that even though you are tired, you can still press on strongly.

When I ran the Boston Marathon in 2014 (a very special year following the bombing), after cresting Heartbreak Hill and with five miles to go, I mentally transported myself to my usual cutdown tempo route back home. I saw myself there, pressing the pace harder with each mile, and mentally tapped into the feelings I've experienced so many times on that route during training. The result was that those last miles were the fastest miles I ran for that marathon, with significant negative split, as I passed other runners who seemed to be standing still. I set my masters personal best that day and managed to draw on all the physical and mental training I had committed to over that long winter training cycle. Using key runs for both mental and physical training allows you to run the race you're ready to run.

Analyze Training Stats Rationally

Today, there is so much technology available to tell you how you're really feeling—your heart rate, oxygen saturation, chronic stress load, recovery markers, power, and so on. Technology is great when you use it for your own purposes rather than letting it dictate your actions and feelings. Analyzing data is also not entirely straightforward. Was my average heart rate for my easy run really that high? It felt easy, but my watch is saying my $\dot{V}O_2$max just dropped a point! My watch is telling me I slept like garbage, but I feel refreshed in the morning—or my watch is telling me I slept great, but I feel exhausted. And then there are those days when I run a long, hard run and while I'm sitting on the couch that evening, my watch tells me that my recovery time has improved or that it's time to get up and move (you lazy couch potato!).

Technology without rational analysis can undermine your training—pushing you to do more when you may need to do less, pushing you to do less when you feel like you can do more, or just missing the whole point of what it is you're trying to do. Looking at training stats requires understanding both the big and small pictures. When analyzing stats, you need to look at general trends over time.

Week after week, you feel strong and do things you once could not fathom, and along the way, there's an occasional bump in the road, but you bounce back fast, physically and mentally. As time presses on and the weeks are crossed off the calendar, it starts getting real. And then you realize you're seven . . . six . . . five weeks out. Taper looms ahead. Then, of course, there's the main event. Suddenly, the stakes are very dire. Now every single run must be perfect, or doom is sure to follow. And though everything is still going well, as it has been, there comes that dreaded day when you have a (gasp!) bad run. Maybe you fail to hit your tempo paces. Or perhaps you hit them, but it feels so hard—harder than it has felt or harder than it should be. Maybe that last long run felt harder than you thought it should feel. And thanks to that one run, you begin to question all those goals you set so many weeks ago. You wonder about the goals you may have refashioned to reflect the progress you've made. With that one run, you forget all the runs where you felt strong, capable, and fast—where the impossible became possible.

That's the thing about human nature, or at least runner nature, when it comes to training and goals and confidence: You often allow a few bad runs to outweigh dozens upon dozens of good runs. You fear that somehow things have taken a turn for the worse. And in one run, on one day, the whole thing is cast into question, and a deep self-doubt sets in. If you can remember the good, the quantity and quality of which far outweigh the bad, then you avoid this unnecessary worry—or worse, nervous anxiety that can actually cause underperformance. You probably know this quote: "She believed she could, and so she did." It's true to a great extent. If you allow one run to undermine your confidence, then this could have a material effect on your training. The training house of cards is held together by the strength of the mind and the will—your heart and your spirit. If you allow the bad to outweigh the good when that is not really what's happening, then it becomes a self-fulfilling prophecy: She believed she couldn't, and so she didn't.

You are not a machine; you are human, and you have good days and bad days. As I recently said to a runner, "This is not as simple as making a car go faster." You are more than matter, and the variables that affect you are numerous and often mysterious. Don't allow the few instances of bad to overshadow the abundance of good, in running or in life.

If you look at your training rationally—if you examine your stats over the course of the training cycle, ask yourself how you honestly feel for the majority of your runs, and understand you are more likely to question your goals as the race gets closer because the stakes feel higher and the time to fix things grows shorter—then you can have an honest conversation with yourself. Sometimes a coach or a more experienced friend can interject a more rational and reasonable assessment of where you are in relation to your goals. But it's also important to acknowledge that this is a natural process, and the first step to pushing this self-defeating tendency aside is to address it and show yourself where your focus might be undermining all the good work you've been doing. And when you do so and see over time that many of your worries were without merit, you become mentally stronger and can file those tough runs away as just that—a tough run.

The mental and emotional side of running is just as, if not more, important as the physical aspect. This journey requires a willingness to listen to yourself, to trust yourself, and to possibly attempt things that scare you or push you in slightly uncomfortable ways. Running can also be a very social activity and presents opportunities to meet a large community of like-minded, active friends. At the same time, it's also very important that you pick the challenges *you* find worthwhile because those are what will keep you pressing ahead every day.

BIBLIOGRAPHY

Alentorn-Geli, E., K. Samuelsson, V. Musahl, C.L. Green, M. Bhandari, and J. Karlsson. 2017. "The Association of Recreational and Competitive Running With Hip and Knee Osteoarthritis: A Systematic Review and Meta-Analysis." *Journal of Orthopaedic and Sports Physical Therapy* 47 (6): 373-90. https://doi.org/10.2519/jospt.2017.7137.

Barnes, Jonathan, ed. *The Complete Works of Aristotle: The Revised Oxford Translation.* Princeton, New Jersey: Princeton University Press, 1995.

Beliard, S., M. Chauveau, T. Moscatiello, F. Cros, F. Ecarnot, and F. Becker. 2015. "Compression Garments and Exercise: No Influence of Pressure Applied." *Journal of Sports Science and Medicine* 14 (1): 75-83. www.ncbi.nlm.nih.gov/pmc/articles/PMC4306786/.

Bosquet, L. and I. Mujika. 2012. "Detraining." In *Endurance Training: Science and Practice*, edited by I. Mujika, 100-106. www.researchgate.net/publication/236590070.

Chaabene, H., D.G. Behm, Y. Negra, and U. Granacher. 2019. "Acute Effects of Static Stretching on Muscle Strength and Power: An Attempt to Clarify Previous Caveats." *Frontiers in Physiology* 10: Article 1468. https://doi.org/10.3389/fphys.2019.01468.

Chakravarty, E.F., H.B. Hubert, V.B. Lingala, and J.F. Fries. 2008. "Reduced Disability and Mortality Among Aging Runners: A 21-Year Longitudinal Study." *Archives of Internal Medicine* 168 (15): 1638-46. https://doi.org/10.1001/archinte.168.15.1638.

Chaput, J.P., C. Dutil, and H. Sampasa-Kanyinga. 2018. "Sleeping Hours: What Is the Ideal Number and How Does Age Impact This?" *Nature and Science of Sleep* 10:421-30. https://doi.org/10.2147/NSS.S163071.

Dąbrowska, J., M. Dąbrowska-Galas, M. Rutkowska, and B.A. Michalski. 2016. "Twelve-Week Exercise Training and the Quality of Life in Menopausal Women: Clinical Trial." *Menopause Review* 15 (1): 20-25. https://doi.org/10.5114/pm.2016.58769.

Dąbrowska-Galas, M., J. Dąbrowska, K. Ptaszkowski, and R. Plinta. 2019. "High Physical Activity Level May Reduce Menopausal Symptoms." *Medicina* 55 (8): 466. https://www.doi.org/10.3390/medicina55080466.

Dalleck, L.C., B.A. Allen, B.A. Hanson, E.C. Borresen, M.E. Erickson, and S.L. De Lap. 2009. "Dose-Response Relationship Between Moderate-Intensity Exercise Duration and Coronary Heart Disease Risk Factors in Postmenopausal Women." *Journal of Women's Health* 18 (1): 105-13. https://doi.org/10.1089/jwh.2008.0790.

Davis, H.L., S. Alabed, and T.J.A. Chico. 2020. "Effect of Sports Massage on Performance and Recovery: A Systematic Review and Meta-Analysis." *BMJ Open Sport and Exercise Medicine* 6 (1): e000614. https://doi.org/10.1136/bmjsem-2019-000614.

Elavsky, S. and E. McAuley. 2007. "Physical Activity and Mental Health Outcomes During Menopause: A Randomized Controlled Trial." *Annals of Behavioral Medicine* 33 (2): 132-42. https://doi.org/10.1007/BF02879894.

Fair, R.C. and E.H. Kaplan. 2018. "Estimating Aging Effects in Running Events." *The Review of Economics and Statistics* 100 (4): https://doi.org/10.1162/rest_a_00725.

Figueroa, A., S.B. Going, L.A. Milliken, R.M. Blew, S. Sharp, P.J. Teixeira, and T.G. Lohman. 2003. "Effects of Exercise Training and Hormone Replacement Therapy on Lean and Fat Mass in Postmenopausal Women." *The Journals of Gerontology: Series A* 58 (3): M266-70. https://doi.org/10.1093/gerona/58.3.M266.

Fries, J.F., G. Singh, D. Morfeld, H.B. Hubert, N.E. Lane, and B.W. Brown. 1994. "Running and the Development of Disability With Age." *Annals of Internal Medicine* 121 (7): 502-9. https://doi.org/10.7326/0003-4819-121-7-199410010-00005.

Frost, H.M. 2000. "The Utah Paradigm of Skeletal Physiology: An Overview of Its Insights for Bone, Cartilage, and Collagenous Tissue Organs." *Journal of Bone and Mineral Metabolism* 18 (6): 305-16. https://doi.org/10.1007/s007740070001.

Fuchs, C.J., I.W.K. Kouw, T.A. Churchward-Venne, J.S.J. Smeets, J.M. Senden, W.D. van Marken Lichtenbelt, L.B. Verdijk, and L.J.C. van Loon. 2020. "Postexercise Cooling Impairs Muscle Protein Synthesis Rates in Recreational Athletes." *Journal of Physiology* 598 (4): 755-72. https://doi.org/10.1113/JP278996.

Gardner, B., P. Lally, and J. Wardle. 2012. "Making Health Habitual: The Psychology of 'Habit-Formation' and General Practice." *British Journal of General Practice* 62 (605): 664-66. https://doi.org/10.3399/bjgp12X659466.

Grant, M.D., A. Marbella, A.T. Wang, E. Pines, J. Hoag, C. Bonnell, K.M. Ziegler, and N. Aronson. 2015. "Menopausal Symptoms: Comparative Effectiveness of Therapies." *Agency for Healthcare Research and Quality (US) Comparative Effectiveness Reviews* 147 (March). www.ncbi.nlm.nih.gov/books/NBK285463/.

Haun, C.T., M.D. Roberts, M.A. Romero, S.C. Osburn, C.B. Mobley, R.G. Anderson, M.D. Goodlett, D.D. Pascoe, and J.S. Martin. 2017. "Does External Pneumatic Compression Treatment Between Bouts of Overreaching Resistance Training Sessions Exert Differential Effects on Molecular Signaling and Performance-Related Variables Compared to Passive Recovery? An Exploratory Study." *PLoS One* 12 (6): e0180429. https://doi.org/10.1371/journal.pone.0180429.

Howden, E.J., S. Sarma, J.S. Lawley, M. Opondo, W. Cornwell, D. Stoller, M.A. Urey, B. Adams-Huet, and B.D. Levine. 2018. "Reversing the Cardiac Effects of Sedentary Aging in Middle Age—A Randomized Controlled Trial: Implications for Heart Failure Prevention." *Circulation* 137 (15): 1549-60. https://doi.org/10.1161/CIRCULATIONAHA.117.030617.

Ji, J., Y. Hou, Z. Li, Y. Zhou, H. Xue, T. Wen, T. Yang, L. Xue, Y. Tu, and T. Ma. 2023. "Association Between Physical Activity and Bone Mineral Density in Postmenopausal Women: A Cross-Sectional Study From the NHANES 2007-2018." *Journal of Orthopaedic Surgery and Research* 18 (501). https://doi.org/10.1186/s13018-023-03976-2.

Jokl, P., P.M. Sethi, and A.J. Cooper. 2004. "Master's Performance in the New York City Marathon 1983-1999." *British Journal of Sports Medicine* 38 (4): 408-12. https://bjsm.bmj.com/content/38/4/408.

Konrad, A., C. Glashüttner, M.M. Reiner, D. Bernsteiner, and M. Tilp. 2020. "The Acute Effects of a Percussive Massage Treatment With a Hypervolt Device on Plantar Flexor Muscles' Range of Motion and Performance." *Journal of Sports Science and Medicine* 19 (4): 690-94. https://pubmed.ncbi.nlm.nih.gov/33239942/.

Leeder, J.D.C., K.A. van Someren, P.G. Bell, J.R. Spence, A.P. Jewell, D. Gaze, and G. Howatson. 2015. "Effects of Seated and Standing Cold Water Immersion on Recovery From Repeated Sprinting." *Journal of Sports Sciences* 33 (15): 1544-52. https://doi.org/10.1080/02640414.2014.996914.

Li, J., M.V. Vitiello, and N. Gooneratne. 2018. "Sleep in Normal Aging." *Sleep Medicine Clinics* 13 (1): 1-11. https://doi.org/10.1016/j.jsmc.2017.09.001.

Lo, G.H., J.B. Driban, A.M. Kriska, T.E. McAlindon, R.B. Souza, N.J. Petersen, K.L. Storti, et al. 2017. "Is There an Association Between a History of Running and Symptomatic Knee Osteoarthritis? A Cross-Sectional Study From the Osteoarthritis Initiative." *Arthritis Care and Research* 69 (2): 183-91. https://doi.org/10.1002/acr.22939.

Lum, D., G. Landers, and P. Peeling. 2010. "Effects of a Recovery Swim on Subsequent Running Performance." *International Journal of Sports Medicine* 31 (1): 26-30. https://doi.org/10.1055/s-0029-1239498.

Marcus, J. 2023. "Older Runners Lacing Up in Greater Numbers." *AARP*. Last modified April 18, 2023. www.aarp.org/health/healthy-living/info-2023/older-runners-on-the-rise.html.

Mikkelsen, U.R., H. Langberg, I.C. Helmark, D. Skovgaard, L.L. Andersen, M. Kjaer, and A.L. Mackey. 2009. "Local NSAID Infusion Inhibits Satellite Cell Proliferation in Human Skeletal Muscle After Eccentric Exercise." *Journal of Applied Physiology* 107 (5): 1600-11. https://doi.org/10.1152/japplphysiol.00707.2009.

Murray, B. and C. Rosenbloom. 2018. "Fundamentals of Glycogen Metabolism for Coaches and Athletes." *Nutrition Reviews* 76 (4): 243-59. https://doi.org/10.1093/nutrit/nuy001.

O'Donnell, S., C.M. Beaven, and M.W. Driller. 2018. "From Pillow to Podium: A Review on Understanding Sleep for Elite Athletes." *Nature and Science of Sleep* 10:243-53. https://doi.org/10.2147/NSS.S158598.

Patoz, A., T. Lussiana, B. Breine, C. Gindre, and K. Hébert-Losier. 2022. "There Is No Global Running Pattern More Economic Than Another at Endurance Running Speeds." *International Journal of Sports Physiology and Performance* 17 (4): 659-62. https://doi.org/10.1123/ijspp.2021-0345.

Pontzer, H., Y. Yamada, H. Sagayama, P.N. Ainslie, L.F. Andersen, L.J. Anderson, L. Arab, et al. 2021. "Daily Energy Expenditure Through the Human Life Course." *Science* 373 (6556): 808-12. https://doi.org/10.1126/science.abe5017.

Sams, L., B.L. Langdown, J. Simons, and J. Vseteckova. 2023. "The Effect of Percussive Therapy on Musculoskeletal Performance and Experiences of Pain: A Systematic Literature Review." *International Journal of Sports Physical Therapy* 18 (2): 309-27. https://doi.org/10.26603/001c.73795.

Stengel, S.V., W. Kemmler, R. Pintag, C. Beeskow, J. Weineck, D. Lauber, W.A. Kalender, and K. Engelke. 2005. "Power Training Is More Effective Than Strength Training for Maintaining Bone Mineral Density in Postmenopausal Women." *Journal of Applied Physiology* 99 (1): 1-380. https://doi.org/10.1152/japplphysiol.01260.2004.

Wiewelhove, T., A. Döweling, C. Schneider, L. Hottenrott, T. Meyer, M. Kellmann, M. Pfeiffer, and A. Ferrauti. 2019. "A Meta-Analysis of the Effects of Foam Rolling on Performance and Recovery." *Frontiers in Physiology* 10 (376). https://doi.org/10.3389/fphys.2019.00376.

INDEX

A

Achilles tendinitis or tendinopathy 89-90
active recovery 69, 107, 127, 158, 159
acute injuries 83-84
adenosine triphosphate (ATP) 13, 64, 67, 188-189
advanced training plans
   for 5K races 129-132
   for marathons 147-152
   for 10K races 132-135
aerobic base 53, 54, 57, 64-72, 143, 171
aerobic running
   foundation of 57
   hill work and 142
   hormonal changes and 42-43
   metabolic system and 69
   progressive overload and 118
   recovery and 100
   tapering and 60, 124, 142
   in training plans 123, 141
   variations in 71-72
age and aging. *See also* older runners
   age grading 30
   athletic age 56-57
   physical changes associated with 11-19
   running and delayed effects of 12
   social and cultural views of 4, 9-11
all-comers meets 163
anabolic hormones 18-19, 38, 40, 77
anti-inflammatory medications 84, 101
Aristotle 5-6, 27, 31, 65, 176
articular cartilage 14
athletic age 56-57
ATP. *See* adenosine triphosphate (ATP)

B

begging the question fallacy 26
beginner training plans
   for 5K races 124-125
   for half-marathons 135-138
   for marathons 143-147
   for 10K races 124-126
Big Sur International Marathon 195
block periodization 52, 53
body composition 18, 38, 40

bone density 14-16, 37, 39-40, 91
bone health 14-16, 39, 41-42, 44
Boston Marathon 172, 195, 198
burnout 62, 99, 107

C

cadence 18, 81, 94
calcium 14-16, 44
carbohydrates 38, 64, 67, 100
cardiac output 16-17
cardiorespiratory fitness 76
carry exercises 78
chronic injuries. *See* overuse injuries
classical (linear) periodization 52, 53
coaches 54, 56, 94, 105, 119, 163, 171
cold-water immersion (CWI) 104
collagen 44, 89
competition phase of macrocycle 51
competitiveness 168
compression clothing 104-105
cortisol 102
CrossFit 64, 117
cross-training
   aerobic base and 64
   benefits of 24, 75
   cycling 76-77, 88
   in detraining cycles 160, 161
   ellipticals 77
   mobility work and 79-80
   rowing exercises 77
   running augmented by 74-80
   strength training 77-79
   swimming and water exercises 75-76, 88, 89, 107
   in training plans 116-117, 123
cutdown runs 123, 141, 198
CWI (cold-water immersion) 104
cycling 76-77, 88

D

data analysis 198-200
delayed-onset muscle soreness (DOMS) 103, 104
detraining cycles 158-162
diet. *See* nutrition

distance running. *See also specific races*
  aerobic base for 64, 65, 68
  human ability/capacity for 6
  injury concerns and 92, 93
  specificity principle and 74
DOMS (delayed-onset muscle soreness) 103, 104
drop of running shoes 82
dynamic stretching 80, 105, 116, 186

E

eating habits. *See* nutrition
elevation changes 190, 191
ellipticals 77
endurance running. *See* distance running
endurance training 42, 52-53, 66-67, 69
estrogen 15, 18, 36, 37-40, 78
eudaemonia 5-6
even splits 187
exercise. *See* training and exercise
external pneumatic compression boots 103

F

fartleks 14, 118, 123, 142
fatigue
  accumulated 53
  sleep quality and 23
  of targeted muscle groups 42
  from too much too soon 113
  training plan adjustments due to 140
fats 38, 64, 66-67, 69, 189
female runners
  counteracting hormone changes in 40-44
  gender stereotypes and 41, 45, 168
  menopause and hormone changes in 36-40
  reasons for avoidance of racing 168
  strength and resistance training for 40-42, 77-78
5K races
  nutrition and 184
  out-of-season cycles 162
  pacing during 187-188
  recovery plans for 158
  training plans for 122-125, 127-132
  warm-ups on race day 186
flexibility 12, 18, 101, 103-104, 115-117
foam rollers 104
food intake. *See* nutrition
foot strike 80-81
footwear 81-83, 86

G

gender stereotypes 41, 45, 168
glycogen 13, 69, 100, 102, 189
goal setting
  alignment with training 54-56
  importance of 171-172
  for older runners 4, 28-31
  process vs. outcome 194-197
  on race day 182-183
  recovery plans and 158
  in training plans 114-115
groupthink 180

H

habit formation 26-28
half-marathons
  nutrition and 184
  out-of-season cycles 163
  pacing during 187-188
  recovery plans for 158, 159
  training plans for 122-124, 135-138
  warm-ups on race day 186
hamstring strains 92-93
happiness 6-7, 31, 32, 36
heart rate 16, 22, 23, 58, 98, 115
HGH. *See* human growth hormone (HGH)
high-intensity interval training (HIIT) 64, 117
hill work 12, 14, 42-43, 52-53, 57, 118, 123, 141-142
hinge exercises 79
hitting the wall 189
hormone replacement therapy (HRT) 44
hormones. *See also specific hormones*
  anabolic 18-19, 38, 40, 77
  bone health and 15
  counteracting changes to 40-44
  menopause and changes to 36-40
  sleep and 13, 19, 44, 102
HRT (hormone replacement therapy) 44
human growth hormone (HGH) 13, 15, 19, 37-38, 44, 102

I

ice baths 104
iliotibial band (ITB) syndrome 90-91
imagery 198
inactivity 11, 13, 17-18, 27-28, 40
inflammation 76, 84, 90, 100, 101, 104
injuries 83-95
  Achilles tendinitis or tendinopathy 89-90

injuries *(continued)*
　acute 83-84
　hamstring strains 92-93
　iliotibial band syndrome 90-91
　minimization of 76, 94-95, 99, 107, 113
　overuse 24, 84, 88
　plantar fasciitis 87-88
　powerlifting and 41
　proximal hamstring tendinopathy 93-94
　risk of 16, 53, 64, 75, 80, 81
　runner's knee 88-89
　shin splints 85-86
　stress fractures 85, 91-92
insertional tendinitis 89, 90
intermediate training plans
　for 5K races 127-129
　for half-marathons 135-138
　for marathons 147-152
　for 10K races 127-129
ITB (iliotibial band) syndrome 90-91

J

James, William 7-8, 11
joint health 14

L

lactate threshold (LT) 69, 158, 178, 188-189, 191
Lewis, C.S. 31
linear (classical) periodization 52, 53
lunges 78-80, 116

M

macrocycles 50-52, 54, 59, 98, 99, 158
mantras 185-186
marathons
　Big Sur 195
　Boston 172, 195, 198
　hitting the wall during 189
　New York City 172, 174-177, 182-183
　out-of-season cycles 162
　pacing during 187-189
　recovery plans for 158, 159
　training plans for 140-152
　warm-ups on race day 186
massage 24, 84, 94, 100-101, 103, 104, 107
massage guns 103
maximal oxygen consumption ($\dot{V}O_2max$) 13, 16
maximal shoes 83
medial tibial stress syndrome (MTSS) 85-86

melatonin 39, 44
menopause 36-40, 44-45
mental health 8, 10, 12, 33, 39, 40
mental imagery 198
mesocycles 50-54, 59, 98, 158
metabolism 18, 38, 66-67, 69, 186
microcycles 50-54, 59, 98
midpoint tendinitis 89, 90
Mill, John Stuart 6-7
minimal shoes 83
mitochondria 13, 65-67
mobility. *See also* range of motion
　aging and 12, 18
　cross-training and 79-80
　explosive exercises for 42
　menopause and 38
　swimming and 75, 76
　warm-ups and 115
MTSS (medial tibial stress syndrome) 85-86
muscle elasticity 115
muscle mass 13-14, 37, 38, 40, 44, 77
muscle soreness 23, 76, 77, 99, 101, 103-104

N

negative splits 186, 198
neutral shoes 83
New York City Marathon (NYCM) 172, 174-177, 182-183
Nietzsche, Friedrich 23
nonsteroidal anti-inflammatory drugs (NSAIDs) 101
nutrition. *See also* proteins
　bone health and 15, 44
　carbohydrates 38, 64, 67, 100
　fats 38, 64, 66-67, 69, 189
　race-day strategies and 183-184
　recovery and 13, 100, 107
　training plans and 117
NYCM. *See* New York City Marathon (NYCM)

O

offseason. *See* out-of-season cycles
older runners. *See also* age and aging; female runners; training and exercise
　finding greatness 31-32
　goal setting for 4, 28-31
　growth in number of 8-9
　habit formation by 26-28
　misconceptions regarding 9
　motivations of 8-10, 26

osteoblasts and osteoclasts 15, 39
osteoporosis and osteopenia 39, 42
out-of-season cycles 51, 105, 162-163
overtraining 50, 62, 88, 101, 103, 115
overuse injuries 24, 84, 88, 101

P

pacing 186-191
pain
    of Achilles tendinitis 89
    anti-inflammatory medications for 101
    chronic 24
    from inactivity 18
    of ITB syndrome 90, 91
    of joints 14
    of plantar fasciitis 87, 88
    of proximal hamstring tendinopathy 93
    of runner's knee 88
    of shin splints 85, 86
    sore muscles 23, 76, 77, 99, 101, 103-104
parkruns 163
passive recovery 76
peaking 54, 60-61
percussive massage devices 103
perimenopause 36-37, 39
periodization 50-54
personal trainers 42, 78, 94
PF (plantar fasciitis) 87-88
physical health 8, 10, 33, 39
physical therapists (PTs) 84, 87, 88, 90, 94
plans for training. *See* training plans
plantar fasciitis (PF) 87-88
plateaus 23-24, 62, 69, 75, 83, 99, 101.
plyometrics 42
positive splits 187
postmenopause 36-40, 44
powerlifting 41
preparation phase of macrocycle 51
press exercises 78
progesterone 39
progression runs 71, 123, 141
progressive overload 50, 86, 113, 115, 118
pronation 83, 86, 90
proteins
    breakdown 38, 64
    intake 13, 38, 44, 100
    synthesis 13, 37, 38, 44, 104
proximal hamstring tendinopathy 93-94
PTs. *See* physical therapists (PTs)
pulling exercises 78
push exercises 78

Q

quality of life 19, 39, 40, 44

R

race-day strategies 182-192
    goal setting and 182-183
    nutrition and 183-184
    pacing and 186-191
    routines and 184-186
    for smart racing 192
    warm-ups and 186
race-pace runs 123, 141
racing 168-180. *See also* race-day strategies; *specific races*
    motivations for 168, 173
    peaking for 54, 60-61
    physiological impacts of 100
    reasons for avoidance of 168-173
    selecting your race 173-180
    social elements of 122, 170, 178
range of motion (ROM). *See also* mobility
    active recovery and 159
    massage/massage guns and 101, 103
    warm-ups and 79-80, 116
Rate of Perceived Effort (RPE) 58
recovery. *See* rest and recovery
recovery boots 103
resistance training. *See* strength and resistance training
responsive training 38, 57-58
rest and recovery 98-107. *See also* sleep
    active recovery 69, 107, 127, 158, 159
    anti-inflammatory medications for 101
    cycling for 77
    massage for 100-101, 103, 104, 107
    during menopause 44
    need for 12-13, 98-100
    nutrition and 13, 100, 107
    passive recovery 76
    planning for 59
    protocols for 100-105
    sleep and 13, 19, 23, 44, 101-103, 107
    swimming for 76
    tools for 103-105
    in training plans 117-118
    transition periods of 51, 105-107, 158-159
resting heart rate 23, 98
rolling massagers 104
ROM. *See* range of motion
rotational exercises 79
rowing exercises 77

RPE (Rate of Perceived Effort) 58
runner's knee 88-89
running. *See also* aerobic running; distance running; female runners; injuries; older runners; racing
   all-comers meets 163
   cadence 18, 81, 94
   creativity in 4, 32, 42
   cross-training as supplement to 74-80
   cutdown runs 123, 141, 198
   economy and efficiency 70
   effects of aging delayed by 12
   motivations for 8-10, 26, 194
   parkruns 163
   progression runs 71, 123, 141
   proper technique for 80-81
   race-pace runs 123, 141
   shakeout runs 124
   shoe considerations 81-83, 86
   social function of 24-25, 122, 200
   sprint-floats 43, 124, 142
   steady-state runs 141
   stride length 18, 43, 94, 122, 140
   tempo runs 66, 100, 123, 141, 163, 178, 184, 187

S

sarcopenia 13
sedentary lifestyle. *See* inactivity
self-belief 197-198
self-care 24, 105
self-fulfilling prophecy 199
serotonin 39
shakeout runs 124
shin splints 85-86
shoes 81-83, 86
shoulder season. *See* out-of-season cycles
sleep
   hormones and 13, 19, 44, 102
   during menopause 37-40, 44
   recovery and 13, 19, 23, 44, 101-103, 107
soles of running shoes 82
specificity of training 64, 68-70, 74
speed work 12-13, 22, 52-54, 57, 60, 118, 124
sprint-floats 43, 124, 142
squats 79, 80
stability shoes 83
stack of running shoes 82
stagnation 50, 70, 114

static stretching 105, 116
steady-state runs 141
stereotypes, gender-based 41, 45, 168
strength and resistance training 14, 15, 40-42, 74, 76-79, 112-113
stress
   adaptation to 13, 14, 23, 37, 114
   anticipatory 163
   bone health and 14-16, 39, 44, 78
   mechanical 14, 15, 39, 76
   overuse injuries and 84
   pain caused by 86
   physical and mental 160
   powerlifting and 41
   recovery and 62, 98, 104
   reduction of 100, 107
   10-percent rule and 52
stress fractures 85, 91-92
stretching 80, 84, 93, 105, 116, 186
stride length 18, 43, 94, 122, 140
swimming 75-76, 88, 89, 107
synovial fluid 14, 18, 115

T

tapering 60, 124, 142
technical demands 190-191
tempo runs 66, 100, 123, 141, 163, 178, 184, 187
10K races
   nutrition and 184
   pacing during 187-188
   recovery plans for 158
   training plans for 122-129, 132-135
   warm-ups on race day 186
10-percent rule 52, 71
tendinitis or tendinopathy 89-90, 93-94
testosterone 15, 18, 37-38, 40
trail shoes 83
training and exercise. *See also* cross-training; rest and recovery; training plans; warm-ups
   alignment with goals 54-56
   data analysis on 198-200
   detraining cycles 158-162
   endurance 42, 52-53, 66-67, 69
   five principles of 57-61
   health benefits of 40
   high-intensity interval 64, 117
   hill work 12, 14, 42-43, 52-53, 57, 118, 123, 141-142
   overtraining 50, 62, 88, 101, 103, 115
   peaking 54, 60-61

periodization and 50-54
personal trainers 42, 78, 94
plyometrics 42
powerlifting 41
progressive and sequential 58-60
progressive overload in 50, 86, 113, 115, 118
responsive 38, 57-58
smart 22-25, 50, 64, 112, 164
specificity of 64, 68-70, 74
speed work 12-13, 22, 52-54, 57, 60, 118, 124
strength and resistance 14, 15, 40-42, 74, 76-79, 112-113
tapering 60, 124, 142
training plans 112-164
  creation of 112-118
  cross-training in 116-117, 123
  doing too much too soon 112-113
  expecting too much too soon 113-114
  for 5K races 122-125, 127-132
  flexibility of 116-117
  goal setting in 114-115
  for half-marathons 122-124, 135-138
  for marathons 140-152
  nutrition and 117
  progressive overload in 118
  rest and recovery in 117-118
  selection of 119-120
  stagnation due to 114
  for 10K races 122-129, 132-135
  transitional 158-164
  for ultramarathons 140-142, 152-156
  warm-ups in 115-116, 122, 140
transitional periods
  detraining cycles 158-162
  out-of-season cycles 51, 105, 162-163
  rest and recovery 51, 105-107, 158-159
  training plans during 158-164

U

ultramarathons
  pacing during 190-191
  recovery plans for 158
  training plans for 140-142, 152-156
use-it-or-lose-it principle 12, 14, 40, 78
Utah paradigm 15, 16

V

vertical gain 190-191
virtues 27, 31
visualization 198
vitamin D 15, 16, 44
vitamin K 15, 44
$\dot{V}O_2$max (maximal oxygen consumption) 13, 16

W

warm-ups
  for plantar fasciitis 87, 88
  on race day 186
  range of motion and 79-80, 116
  in training plans 115-116, 122, 140
water exercises 75-76
weather considerations 190
winner-takes-all mentality 10
Wolff's law 14-16
women. *See* female runners

ABOUT THE AUTHOR

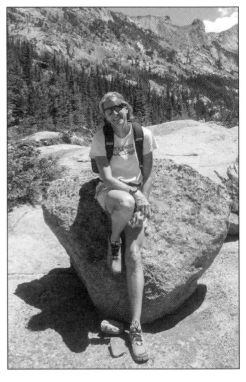

Caolan MacMahon has been dedicated to running since she was eight years old, and she continues to pursue her passion several decades later. She has completed more than 80 marathons and ultramarathons since turning 50, including six Boston Marathons and three New York City Marathons. MacMahon is the 2013 RRCA Grand Master 50K champion and has achieved dozens of overall podium and age-group finishes. She is the head coach and director of The Long Run Coaching LLC. She holds certifications from UESCA (Ultrarunning Coach; Endurance Sports Nutrition Certification), NASM (CPT), World Athletics (Elite L5), USATF (L3 Endurance, Youth Specialization; L2 Endurance/Speed/Hurdles/Relays, Youth Specialization), RRCA, and Lydiard (LI and LII). MacMahon is also a USATF L1 coaching instructor and is a coach and clinician at the USATF youth cross country camp at the Olympic Training Center in Colorado Springs.

Beyond her accomplishments in running and coaching, MacMahon is an educator, rock climber, former professor of philosophy, ethicist, animal activist, and writer. She has been a contributing writer for *Runner's World* and provided race reports and contributions to *Self*, *New York Times*, *Ultra Running Magazine*, *Colorado Runner*, *5280*, and *Elevation Outdoors*. She has also been blogging for *The Chronic Runner* since 2011.